T0212421

Developing a Program
of Research in Nursing

Cheryl Tatano Beck, DNSc, CNM, FAAN, is a distinguished professor at the University of Connecticut School of Nursing. She also has a joint appointment in the Department of Obstetrics and Gynecology at the School of Medicine. Her bachelor of science degree in nursing is from Western Connecticut State University. She received her master's degree in maternal–newborn nursing from Yale University. Dr. Beck holds a certificate in nurse-midwifery, also from Yale University. Her doctor of nursing science degree is from Boston University. She is a fellow in the American Academy of Nursing and has received numerous awards, including the Association of Women's Health, Obstetric, and Neonatal Nursing's Distinguished Professional Service Award; the Eastern Nursing Research Society's Distinguished Researcher Award; the Distinguished Alumna Award from Yale University; and the Connecticut Nurses' Association's Diamond Jubilee Award for her contribution to nursing research. She has been appointed to the President's Advisory Council of Postpartum Support International.

Over the past 30 years, Dr. Beck has focused her research efforts on developing a research program on postpartum mood and anxiety disorders. Based on the findings from her series of qualitative studies, she developed the Postpartum Depression Screening Scale (PDSS), which is published by Western Psychological Services. She is a prolific writer who has published over 140 journal articles covering such topics as phenomenology, grounded theory, narrative analysis, metasynthesis, and qualitative secondary analysis. She is coauthor, with Dr. Denise Polit, of the textbook *Nursing Research: Generating and Assessing Evidence for Nursing Practice*. Editions of this text received both the 2007 and the 2011 *American Journal of Nursing (AJN)* Book of the Year Award. Their *Essentials of Nursing Research* textbook won the 2013 *AJN* Book of the Year Award. Dr. Beck coauthored, with Dr. Jeanne Driscoll, *Postpartum Mood and Anxiety Disorders: A Clinician's Guide*, which received the 2006 *AJN* Book of the Year Award. Her recent books include *Traumatic Childbirth* and *The Routledge International Handbook of Qualitative Nursing Research*.

Developing a Program of Research in Nursing

Cheryl Tatano Beck, DNSc, CNM, FAAN

SPRINGER PUBLISHING COMPANY

NEW YORK

Springer Publishing Company, LLC
11 West 42nd Street
New York, NY 10036
www.springerpub.com

Acquisitions Editor: Joseph Morita
Production Editor: Kris Parrish
Composition: S4Carlisle Publishing Services

ISBN: 978-0-8261-2325-1
e-book ISBN: 978-0-8261-2326-8

15 16 17 18 / 5 4 3 2 1

The author and the publisher of this Work have made every effort to use sources believed to be reliable to provide information that is accurate and compatible with the standards generally accepted at the time of publication. Because medical science is continually advancing, our knowledge base continues to expand. Therefore, as new information becomes available, changes in procedures become necessary. We recommend that the reader always consult current research and specific institutional policies before performing any clinical procedure. The author and publisher shall not be liable for any special, consequential, or exemplary damages resulting, in whole or in part, from the readers' use of, or reliance on, the information contained in this book. The publisher has no responsibility for the persistence or accuracy of URLs for external or third-party Internet websites referred to in this publication and does not guarantee that any content on such websites is, or will remain, accurate or appropriate.

Library of Congress Cataloging-in-Publication Data

Beck, Cheryl Tatano, author.
 Developing a program of research in nursing / Cheryl Tatano Beck.
    p. ; cm.
 Includes bibliographical references and index.
 ISBN 978-0-8261-2325-1 — ISBN 978-0-8261-2326-8 (eISBN)
 I. Title.
 [DNLM: 1. Nursing Research. 2. Program Development—methods. 3. Research Design. WY 20.5]
 RT81.5
 610.73072—dc23
                                                                                    2015032102

Printed in the United States of America by McNaughton & Gunn.

To my mother, who instilled in me during early childhood the importance of education and a strong work ethic in order to succeed in life.

Contents

Preface

In today's academic world, there is nothing more important for a nurse researcher than to develop a systematic program of research. A valuable research trajectory is needed not only for promotion and tenure in your own academic career, but also for the discipline of nursing and for improvements in patient care. In helping my PhD students over the years to start to plan their own research trajectories, I often wished there had been a textbook I could direct them to for guidance on the ins and outs of developing a program of research. There were many books on how to write successful grant proposals. However, not being able to find a book specifically addressing the question of developing a research program became my impetus to embark on writing it myself. I wrote the book for the benefit of not only my own PhD students, but all PhD students, as well as for junior faculty new to the academic world.

I wanted to share with beginning nurse researchers what I have learned while immersed in my own research program for the past 30 years. I guess if someone asked me to identify the best pearl of wisdom I could share regarding a program of research, it would have to be that a truly valuable research program for a discipline is knowledge driven and not method limited. Gone are the days when a nurse researcher would have a program of research that was totally quantitative or qualitative. As you journey along your research path, what is most exciting is just where that path will lead you. Will your next study be qualitative? Quantitative? Or mixed methods? You cannot predict the direction your program of research will take as you start your journey. Trust me, you will never be bored developing your research trajectory. Unforeseen challenges await you, for example, as you cross over from completing a quantitative research study to your first qualitative study now, or vice versa.

As I began my program of research, I never, for instance, envisioned that years later I would be involved in instrument development; but, indeed, that is where my research path led me. I went on to develop the Postpartum Depression Screening Scale, not only in English but also in Spanish. At first, I was hesitant to take on instrument development as my next study in my research trajectory, even though that was where the state of the knowledge at that time on screening for postpartum depression was leading me.

Not having had an instrument development course in my doctoral program at Boston University, I knew I needed to consult with a psychometrician. Do not be afraid to use consultants in your research program. You are not expected to be an expert in every type of research design. A warning, though: Take your time deciding on a consultant. Review the curricula vitae (CVs) of potential consultants. Look at their track records with grants and publications. Obtain copies of articles they have written to assess the rigor of the method for which you are interested in consulting with them. In my case, the time I devoted to choosing a consultant to guide me in developing and testing the Postpartum Depression Screening Scale was one of the best investments in time that I have made in my program of research. I decided on Robert Gable, EdD, and we have since collaborated for the past 20 years.

In the beginning of my research program, phenomenology was the qualitative research design with which I felt most comfortable, and so I began with that design. I expanded my series of qualitative studies from just using a phenomenological design to using grounded theory and then to narrative analysis. Secondary qualitative data analysis came into play next in my research trajectory. Lastly, in my program of research, my path led me to mixed-methods research for the first time. You are never too old to learn new research designs, if that is where your research program is leading you.

What I have found incredibly helpful in moving my program of research along through the years at a faster pace is to always work on more than one study at a time and write more than one manuscript at a time. Juggling multiple projects prevents you from wasting valuable time. For example, at times you may have to wait to get your research proposal through institutional review boards (IRBs) at different institutions. If you are conducting another study while waiting for these approvals, you can devote your energies to that. Another example focuses on writing up manuscripts from your research. Sometimes, you may get writer's block or just be tired of working on a particular manuscript. If you have another manuscript to work on, you can take a break from the manuscript you are tired of and concentrate on the other one. You can go back and forth between the two manuscripts and make the most of your time.

Throughout this book, I use examples of specific studies from my own research program on postpartum mood and anxiety disorders to illustrate points I am making. These concrete examples are included to help encourage researchers to develop their own research trajectories. I have also included throughout this book the successful and valuable research programs of other nurse researchers to provide more examples in other topic areas besides postpartum mood and anxiety disorders.

The rest of this preface presents an overview of this book and what each of the chapters addresses. In Chapter 1, "Developing a Program of Research," various definitions of a research program are presented along with metaphors used to describe research trajectories. In this chapter, I introduce my own program of research on postpartum mood and anxiety disorders.

In Chapter 2, "Starting a Program of Research," I share my belief that a successful program of research needs to be knowledge driven and not method limited. I introduce the metaphor of paths that I use throughout this book to illustrate points I am making about developing a valuable research program. Next, the tools needed to develop a valuable program of research are described, which include types of successful minds and personality traits needed to achieve this goal. Also addressed is how, in beginning a research program, one gets the ideas for one's research studies. I share my ideas for my studies in my investigation of postpartum mood and anxiety disorders. The chapter ends with examples of other nurse researchers' ideas for their programs of research.

Chapter 3, "Planning Sequential Studies," focuses on providing researchers with illustrations from the sequence of studies in my own research program on postpartum mood and anxiety disorders. Also, the benefits of incorporating meta-analyses and metasyntheses in helping to plan for sequential studies in a research trajectory are discussed. Lastly, the suggestions of seasoned nurse researchers provide valuable guidance in planning sequential studies with special populations.

In Chapter 4, "Options Available for Developing a Research Program," I discuss some of the options other than the usual quantitative research methods to expand the paths that researchers have available to them. The benefits of qualitative research in developing a research program are first discussed. The use of qualitative research in instrument development, in secondary qualitative analysis, in grounded theory modification, and in intervention studies is addressed, as well. For years, researchers have been using the Internet to gather data for their quantitative studies. Options for collecting qualitative data via the Internet are now available and can have numerous benefits for researchers. In the latter part of this chapter, mixed-methods research is presented as another valuable option for researchers in developing programs of research. Examples from my own research trajectory are used to illustrate some of these benefits of qualitative and mixed-methods options.

In Chapter 5, "Sustaining a Program of Research," characteristics of a sustained research trajectory and the steps needed to achieve one are addressed. Also, the benefits of international and intra/interdisciplinary research teams to help move along a program of research are discussed. Collaboration can be key to helping speed your travel down the paths of your research program. Examples of three nurse researchers who have successful collaborative research programs are presented to illustrate intradisciplinary and interdisciplinary research teams.

The programs of research of other nurse researchers are the focus of Chapter 6, in which I have highlighted five successful research programs.

These programs focus on pediatric oncology, marginalized groups, suffering, fatigue, and adult oncology.

The final chapter, Chapter 7, is titled "Publishing Your Program of Research." If a program of research is to provide new discoveries for evidence-based practice, dissemination of its findings is a critical step. This chapter focuses on the challenges of writing and publishing the studies in your research program.

Cheryl Tatano Beck

O · N · E

Developing a Program of Research

A well-beaten path does not always make the right road.
—Proverb

DEFINITIONS OF A PROGRAM OF RESEARCH

In developing a program of research, Eisner (1991) likens it to preparing a fine meal: A "model of knowledge accumulation is less like making deposits to a bank account than preparing a fine meal. Indeed, a fine meal is much more apt an image than either the tidy rationality of a bank account or the redolence of a garbage dump. In a meal, each course connects with and complements the others" (p. 211).

In Table 1.1 are examples of selected definitions of a program of research. All these definitions reflect Eisner's (1998) preparation of a fine meal where each course is connected and complements the others. My own definition of a research program that provides the foundation for this book is as follows: A program of research is a sustained, systematically planned series of studies addressing a particular gap in the knowledge base of a discipline that is knowledge driven and not method limited. Each successive study, complete in itself, builds on previous studies and results in a logical progression of knowledge to fill the identified gap.

The backbone of my perspective in developing a valuable research program for a discipline, such as nursing, is that it is knowledge driven and not method limited. At each juncture, the progression of a program of research can take many different paths. The researcher may need to change from inductive to deductive methods or vice versa. In a research trajectory, there are times when perhaps neither a qualitative nor a quantitative design alone will be the type of design a researcher needs to adequately answer the research

1

• TABLE 1.1 Definitions of a Research Program

Author (Year)	Definition
Pranulis (1991)	A series of related studies aimed at addressing a particular knowledge gap that is significant to the scientist's discipline.
Fitch (1996)	A series of studies conducted in a topic area such that logical progression of knowledge is revealed.
Sandelowski (1997)	Comprising planned, purposeful, and substantive and/or theoretically linked studies with demonstrable significance for the public welfare.
Parse (2009)	Visible testimony demonstrating a coherent pattern of knowledge development about a particular phenomenon.
Holzemer (2009)	Designed to build knowledge over time that can contribute to improved outcomes of health care. It is grounded theoretically and is linked to rigorous research methodologies.
Morse (2010)	Addresses a large programmatic aim, and consists of a series of planned, interrelated, interconnected projects, each complete in itself, and each contributing stepwise to meeting the overall aim.
Social Sciences & Humanities Research Council (Canada) (2013)	A sustained research enterprise that includes one or more projects or other components, and is shaped by broad objectives for the advancement of knowledge. It might be undertaken primarily by one investigator and encompassed within a single research career, or it might mobilize a team of researchers during a specific period.

question. A mixed methods design may be the correct path. The sequence of studies in a program of research is not fixed ahead of time.

There are two common assumptions about qualitative research that can harm a program of research. The first assumption is that qualitative research is a jumping off point in a research program that is followed by quantitative research studies, and the second is that qualitative methods should be used only with a topic area where not much is known or until hypotheses are ready to be tested. Neither of these assumptions is true, and both are based on the mistaken notion that qualitative research is not as rigorous or as valuable as quantitative research. It is the job of the researcher to let the research lead the way, regardless of the method by which it starts or which method will continue the program of research in the most valuable way.

WHO DOES A PROGRAM OF RESEARCH?

Certainly, a research trajectory is essential for nurses in academia. Promotion and tenure are critically tied to demonstration of a research program, especially for nursing faculty at a research-extensive university. It is not enough to conduct a number of different research studies for promotion and tenure. Jumping around from topic to topic, even though these topics are relevant to your discipline, will not be nearly enough to achieve tenure. The research studies must focus on the same topic area and be linked together in order to develop a valuable program of research. Nurses in academia are not the only ones conducting studies. There are positions in health care agencies for nurse researchers. Not only researchers but also the discipline of nursing benefits from a sustained research program. Research programs provide a strong foundation for evidence-based practice.

METAPHORS USED TO DESCRIBE RESEARCH PROGRAMS

Kangas, Warren, and Byrne (1998) conducted a secondary qualitative data analysis of nurse researchers' narratives describing their research programs. Metaphors were frequently used to describe the development of their research trajectories. These narratives revealed metaphors of growth, building, sports, and violence. Several researchers used growth-related metaphors to describe their research journey. One nurse researcher compared hers to a growth process that starts with one idea, which leads to another, and to another, and so on. She likened this to a tree trunk with a number of branches. Another nurse researcher explained the helpfulness of a number of small studies to grow a program of research. She urged new researchers not to get discouraged if they were not successful in securing large grants at the beginning.

Building was another frequently used metaphor by the participants; for instance, "So that what you're doing is you're just laying it brick by brick on the foundation" (Kangas et al., 1998, p. 192). One study builds on another one.

As other nurse researchers described their progression through their research trajectories, sports metaphors were utilized. One researcher talked about funding agencies that are interested in whether a person has a track record of successful research. Another participant in Kangas and colleagues' study described having a person on your research team who is inside the clinical agency where you want to collect your data. Visualizing a successful program of research as teamwork was another sports metaphor used.

The last group of metaphors that Kangas and colleagues (1998) identified in their secondary data analysis reflected *violent* metaphors of burning and drowning. One nurse researcher felt like she was drowning in data. An example of the burning metaphor was illustrated by the following quote:

> It was the first research grant, and it was hell. You know, managing the budget and data and all of those things you didn't even know you needed to worry about. Data entry, data cleaning, all that. I didn't have help. Grants were small. It was all on my back. I had to do it all. So by the time I finished the second one . . . I was really burned out on grants management. (Kangas et al., 1998, p. 192)

The metaphors of growth and building reflect journeys that were more sequential and hierarchical in nature, while the sports and violence metaphors bring out the competitive nature of research programs.

MY PROGRAM OF RESEARCH

My program of research began in the early 1980s after I had received my doctorate in nursing from Boston University. As a nurse-midwife, I saw firsthand how devastating postpartum depression was for new mothers. When I went to the medical and nursing textbooks to learn more about this postpartum mood disorder, all I could find in the early 1980s were a few short sentences describing symptoms. It was then that I decided to dedicate my research career to studying postpartum mood and anxiety disorders.

My courses at Boston University were all focused on quantitative research design methods and statistics. In the late 1970s and early 1980s, qualitative research courses in nursing doctoral programs were rarities. Armed as I was with only quantitative research courses, my first study after my receiving my doctorate was what I knew best—a quantitative research design. I blended my dissertation topic of temporal experiences with postpartum depression. After completing this quantitative study where I measured mothers' postpartum depressive symptoms with a general depression scale, I realized I now needed to add mothers' voices and perspectives to the scores on that quantitative instrument. So for my second study after receiving my doctoral degree, I turned to qualitative research methods and my first descriptive phenomenological study of postpartum depression. Because I had no formal courses on qualitative methods, I surrounded myself with not only qualitative research textbooks but the primary sources for each of the qualitative research designs, for example, Colaizzi (1978) for descriptive phenomenology and Husserl's (1931) philosophy that underpins descriptive phenomenology. I cannot stress enough the importance of reading primary sources for the specific qualitative methods you are considering using in your own research program. Currently, there are many qualitative studies published in peer-reviewed journals that used sloppy qualitative methods.

I would like to share two quotes that have made a significant impression on me in my continued drive not to be method limited in my research career but instead to include both qualitative and quantitative methods. The first is a quote by Patton (1990, p. 132): "Qualitative data can put flesh on the bones of quantitative results, bringing the results to life through in depth case elaboration." An example from my program of research illustrating this important point involves a meta-analysis of 19 studies that I conducted (Beck, 1995) to determine the magnitude of the effect of postpartum depression on maternal–infant interaction during the first year after birth. Results revealed that postpartum depression had a large adverse effect on maternal–infant interaction. In the quantitative studies that were included in the meta-analysis, researchers videotaped the mothers interacting with their infants and then coded the videotapes. These researchers often ended their reports almost chastising depressed mothers for failing to respond to their infants' cues. Upon completing this meta-analysis, I reviewed the literature to see if any qualitative studies had been conducted to reveal the mothers' side of these stories. None had been published, so my next study in my research program was a phenomenological study to investigate postpartum depressed mothers' experiences interacting with their infants during the first year after birth (Beck, 1996). The first mother I interviewed began with the following quote. It is my best example of qualitative research putting flesh on the bones of the quantitative findings from my meta-analysis:

> My husband and son got back from the store. I think my 3-year-old son wanted to tell me about something that had happened. It was physically so hard to listen that I really remember just trying to put up some kind of wall so that I wouldn't be battered to death. At this point I was really sitting on the couch trying to figure out whether I could ever move again, and I started to cry. My son started hitting me with his fists and he said "Where are you, Mom?" It was really painful because I didn't have a clue as to where I was either. He was really trying to wake something up, but it was just too far gone. There was no way that I could retrieve the mom that he remembered and hoped he would find, let alone the mother I wanted to be for my new baby. (Beck, 1996, p. 98)

The second quote that supports the value of adding qualitative data to quantitative findings in a research program is one from Selikoff (1991, p. 26): "Statistics are human beings with the tears wiped away." In order to investigate a complete picture of a topic under study, the tears need to be added. One of the best examples of this is from my mixed methods study on secondary traumatic stress in labor and delivery nurses (Beck & Gable, 2012).

The quantitative strand revealed that 35% of the labor and delivery nurses reported moderate to severe levels of secondary traumatic stress resulting from caring for women who had traumatic childbirths. The quote that follows from the qualitative strand of the mixed methods study adds the tears of the nurses to this startling statistic:

> Each traumatic birth adds another scar to my soul. Sometimes I tell my husband that I feel like the picture of Dorian Grey. Somewhere my real face is in a closet and it reveals the awful things I've seen during my labor and delivery career. The face I show the world is of an aging woman who works in this lovely place called a delivery room where happy things happen. (Beck & Gable, 2012, p. 756)

Throughout the remaining chapters of this book, I expand on my postpartum mood and anxiety disorder research program to illustrate points about how to develop a successful and valuable research trajectory.

REFERENCES

Beck, C. T. (1995). The effect of postpartum depression of maternal-infant interaction: A meta-analysis. *Nursing Research, 44*, 298–304.

Beck, C. T. (1996). Postpartum depressed mothers' experiences interacting with their children. *Nursing Research, 45*(2), 98–104.

Beck, C. T., & Gable, R. K. (2012). A mixed methods study of secondary traumatic stress in labor and delivery nurses. *Journal of Obstetric, Gynecologic, and Neonatal Nursing, 41*, 747–760.

Colaizzi, P. E. (1978). Psychological research as the phenomenologist views it. In R. Valle & M. Kings (Eds.), *Existential phenomenological alternatives for psychology* (pp. 48–71). New York, NY: Oxford University Press.

Eisner, E. W. (1998). *The enlightened eye: Qualitative inquiry and the enhancement of educational practice.* New York, NY: Macmillan.

Fitch, I. M. (1996). Creating a research agenda with relevance to cancer nursing practice. *Cancer Nursing, 19*(5), 335–342.

Holzemer, W. L. (2009). Building a program of research. *Japan Journal of Nursing Science, 6*, 1–5.

Husserl, E. (1931). *Ideas: General introduction to pure phenomenology.* New York, NY: Collier Books.

Kangas, S., Warren, N. A., & Byrne, M. M. (1998). Metaphor: The language of nursing researchers. *Nursing Research, 47*(3), 190–193.

Morse, J. M. (2010). What happened to research programs? *Qualitative Health Research, 20*(2), 147.

Parse, R. R. (2009). Knowledge development and programs of research. *Nursing Science Quarterly, 22*, 5–6.

Patton, M. Q. (1990). *Qualitative evaluation and research methods.* Newbury Park, CA: SAGE.

Pranulis, M. F. (1991). Research programs in a clinical setting. *Western Journal of Nursing Research, 13,* 274–277.

Sandelowski, M. J. (1997). Programmatic qualitative research or, appreciating the importance of gas station pumps. In J. M. Morse (Ed.), *Completing a qualitative project: Details and dialogue* (pp. 211–225). Thousand Oaks, CA: SAGE.

Selikoff, I. J. (1991). Asbestos disease 1990–2020: The risks of asbestos risk assessment. *Toxicology and Industrial Health, 7,* 117–126.

Starting a Program of Research

To be a star, you must shine your own light, follow your
own path, and don't worry about the darkness, for that is
when the stars shine brightest.

—Anonymous

When developing a program of research, my mind always comes back to
two poems that reflect my perspective on this long career process. The first is
Robert Frost's famous poem:

THE ROAD NOT TAKEN

Two roads diverged in a yellow wood,
And sorry I could not travel both
And be one traveler, long I stood
And looked down one as far as I could
To where it bent in the undergrowth;
Then took the other, as just as fair,
And having perhaps the better claim,
Because it was grassy and wanted wear;
Though as for that the passing there
Had worn them really about the same,
And both that morning equally lay
In leaves no step had trodden black.
Oh, I kept the first for another day!
Yet knowing how way leads on to way,
I doubted if I should ever come back.

I shall be telling this with a sigh
Somewhere ages and ages hence;
Two roads diverged in a wood, and I
I took the one less traveled by,
And that has made all the difference.
                    —*Robert Frost (1874–1963)*

The second poem is not as well known. It was written by Sam Walter Foss:

THE CALF-PATH

One day, through the primeval wood,
A calf walked home, as good calves should;
But made a trail all bent askew,
A crooked trail, as all calves do.
Since then three hundred years have fled,
And, I infer, the calf is dead.
But still he left behind his trail,
And hereby hangs my moral tale.
The years passed on in swiftness fleet.
The road became a village street,
And this, before men were aware,
A city's crowded thoroughfare,
And soon the central street was this
Of a renowned metropolis;
And men two centuries and a half
Trod in the footsteps of that calf.
Each day a hundred thousand rout
Followed that zigzag calf about,
And o'er his crooked journey went
The traffic of a continent.
A hundred thousand men were led
By one calf near three centuries dead.
They follow still his crooked way,
And lose one hundred years a day,
For thus such reverence is lent
To well-established precedent.
A moral lesson this might teach,
Were I ordained and called to preach;
For men are prone to go it blind

Along the calf-paths of the mind,
And work away from sun to sun
To do what other men have done.
They follow in the beaten track,
And out and in, and forth and back.
And still their devious course pursue,
To keep the path that others do.
They keep the path a sacred groove,
Along which all their lives they move,
But how the wise old wood-gods laugh,
Who saw the first primeval calf!
Ah! Many things this tale might teach
But I am not ordained to preach.
                    —*Sam Walter Foss (1858–1911)*

These poems support the belief that a research program should be knowledge driven and not method limited. When a research trajectory is method limited, it may not be as productive and valuable to a discipline, such as nursing, as when it is driven by the current state of knowledge in that substantive topic and the research questions that beg to be answered at that point in time. What I mean by method limited is staying with either qualitative or quantitative methods throughout your research program because that method is what you are most comfortable with. In a method-limited research program, the researcher may keep choosing the trodden path, the beaten path that keeps that path a "sacred groove." The researcher never goes back to travel the road not taken. One's choice of a path leads to other forks in the road, and so on.

Researchers are not expected to have expertise in all quantitative and qualitative research designs, but that should not prevent them from taking a path different from their previous trodden path. Collaboration with another researcher who has the expertise you are lacking is one option. Budgets in grants can be targeted for needed consultation for the method you are not comfortable with. Mentors, consultants, workshops, and so on, are available to help you gain the needed expertise.

No matter at what point you are in your research trajectory—early, midcareer, or late—you cannot accurately predict what future direction your program of inquiry will take. Each successive study should be guided by the previous research studies. The aim of this systematic, continuous inquiry is the cumulative production of new knowledge in a substantive area. Once the researcher's latest study is completed, then he or she knows the most appropriate path to take for the next study. The current state of knowledge on the research topic and the findings from the researcher's most recently completed project help determine whether the next step in the program of research will lead down a quantitative path, a qualitative path, or perhaps a mixed methods path. Once that is decided, the specific type of quantitative, qualitative, or mixed methods research design is the next decision to be made.

Throughout this book, I use the metaphor of paths to illustrate points I am making about developing a research program. A path is defined as "(1) a trodden track or way, (2) a road, way, or track made for a particular purpose, (3) the route or course along which something travels or moves, and (4) a course of action or conduct" (www.thefreedictionary.com/path). Kroeker warns that "it is not easy to navigate new paths. The familiarity, ease, and convenience of the old paths make them the most likely to take. You may need to do hard work forming new paths in your forest, resisting the urge to take the old familiar ones" (Kroeker, 2008). Venturing out to follow a path of a qualitative study when you are primarily a quantitative researcher (or vice versa) may require the hard work that Kroeker is talking about, but the benefits can be invaluable in a research program.

White's (1998) book, *Paths and Walkways: Simple Projects, Contemporary Designs,* provided the backdrop for my use of paths as the metaphor in developing a program of research. Inside the front cover of White's book is written "In *Paths and Walkways,* Hazel White shows how to create a marvelous garden that invites all who enter to linger, stroll, and unwind in sundappled luxury. Unlike most garden books you have seen, this one does not just make you yearn for the beautiful gardens pictured—it explains exactly how to achieve them yourself, with step-by-step instructions, lists of tools and materials, notes on maintenance, estimated costs, and location tips."

This book focuses on how to create a successful research program that invites clinicians to "linger and stroll" within their research trajectory to provide them with evidence to use in their clinical practice. The chapters that follow provide step-by-step instructions, needed "tools and materials," examples of successful programs, and helpful hints to achieve a valuable program of research.

White (1998) stated that "Paths throw the garden open to exploration. They set people into motion" (p. 7). Just as in a garden, paths at each step in a program of research open it up to exploration by researchers as they deliberate which path to choose at the next fork in the road. Just as paths give structure to a garden, so do they structure research programs. "The paths, the bones, are vital because they organize the space, lead people into and through it, from one area to the next" (White, 1998, p. 11). Every individual's research program will develop differently. For some scientists, their research trajectory will follow a direct path while others' paths may be less direct.

White (1998) described a hierarchy of paths, for not all paths are equal. "Paths that meander for no reason immediately register on the mind as irritating" (p. 15). Paths can be categorized from simple to complex. "The ones categorized as moderately difficult merely contain more steps than the others, or require more attention to detail or a certain level of confidence. If you have never handled a brick or a trowel, there is no need to summon false courage; some of the recipes that are simple and least expensive to build are also the most beautiful" (White, 1998, p. 9). In a research program, if a researcher has never conducted specific research designs (e.g., grounded theory), "there's no need to summon false courage." Collaboration with experts nationally or internationally for that particular research design is one option.

For researchers who have not conducted qualitative research before, Morse (2005) warns of detrimental assumptions, such as the following, to avoid regarding qualitative methods: (a) "There is a clear link between qualitative and quantitative research," (b) "knowing quantitative research helps you learn and/or understand qualitative," and (c) "quantitative researchers can learn qualitative research simply by trying it" (p. 1004). Researchers who subscribe to these erroneous assumptions do not understand that qualitative inquiry is based on an entirely new way of thinking. Qualitative inquiry is not a modification of quantitative research. But do not be discouraged; there are ample resources for learning qualitative inquiry. Doctoral programs offer courses in qualitative methods. Workshops and online courses are available. Grants can be obtained for hiring consultants for the specific type of qualitative design your path is leading you to, such as narrative inquiry or phenomenology.

In an editorial in *Qualitative Health Research,* Morse (2010) asked, "Whatever happened to research programs?" She reported that the most frequent phrase now seen in manuscripts is, "'This work is a part of a larger project'. . . Apparently these researchers are working on something grand, but have decided to throw us some crumbs from the banquet table" (p. 147). "Research program" seems to have been discarded as a descriptor. Articles are published that are related to other studies by the researcher, but readers are not told how, where, or why. Morse proposes that we return to using the term "research program" and only publish articles of planned, self-contained studies that include logic models to illustrate how the studies fit together.

In their doctoral programs, beginning nurse researchers take formal courses on research design, the conduct of individual studies, and grantsmanship. Conn (2004), however, pointed out that less common is the preparation of doctoral students on how to develop a program of research, which is also needed to move the science of our discipline forward and to have successful research careers. There are so many books already published on successful grant writing that this component of a research program is not the focus of this book.

The ideal point of entry for a program of research is during doctoral studies. The dissertation should, hopefully, be the starting and jumping off point for new PhDs in their lifelong journey related to their research program. Other points of entry are possible. For some PhDs, once they have completed their doctoral program, they may take a break from conducting research and decide to focus on their new teaching role as they accept faculty positions at universities. Before they know it, years can pass without any research. Now, however, they are ready to embark on their program of research. Not all PhDs choose academia for their careers. Others may have careers in the clinical area. An example of this career path is PhDs who are employed by health care agencies as nurse researchers to help move along nursing research in those institutions, as a step toward achieving agnet status.

TOOLS NEEDED FOR DEVELOPING A PROGRAM OF RESEARCH

Before we get into some specifics about developing a program of research, let us look more generally at the five types of minds a successful researcher needs and also at the necessary "tools" to achieve one's goals.

Five Minds for the Future

Gardner (2008) proposed five types of minds that an individual needs to succeed in the 21st century. Gardner did not specifically apply his five minds for the future to developing a successful program of research, but, as you will see, this can easily be applied to nurse researchers. His five minds for the future include the disciplined mind, the synthesizing mind, the creating mind, the respectful mind, and the ethical mind. Persons need to have expertise in a discipline and to be able to succinctly put together information from different sources. Persons need to think out of the box and be creative. Also important is being respectful of all persons, not only those who are different but also those who are similar. Lastly, individuals need to be ethical in their actions and do what is right and consider human values. Being ethical involves thinking beyond our own needs to those of others.

Let us look at each mind in a little more depth to visualize how each is necessary for a successful research program. First, in the disciplined mind, an individual has mastered a way of thinking that is characteristic of a specific scholarly discipline or profession. For us, this discipline is nursing. Gardner (2008) cites four steps that are essential to achieve a disciplined mind:

1. You need to identify important topics or concepts within your discipline. Certainly for nurse researchers, a valuable program of research for our discipline starts with the choice of a clinically important topic on which the trajectory will focus.

2. You need to invest significant amounts of time in studying this topic. A successful research trajectory should span a nurse researcher's career and focus on the same topic. Researching different topics will not yield a valuable program of research.

3. You need to approach the topic from many different ways. Applying this step to a research program, nurse researchers should be using both qualitative and quantitative methods to examine their topic.

4. Gardner's fourth step involves setting up a "performance of understanding" (p. 34). This step can be applied to senior researchers who mentor junior faculty just starting out on their research trajectories. Gardner purports that to enhance understanding, it is not enough to determine whether someone understands what was taught since that person may simply be relying on memory. To determine whether understanding has truly been achieved, you need to present the person with a new question or puzzle.

A person with a disciplined mind learns the necessary habits and skills to make steady and continual progress toward his or her goals. Gardner (2008) proposed that disciplined persons continue to learn because they are lifelong learners and have a passion for learning.

The synthesizing mind is also needed for nurse researchers throughout a trajectory of research. The ability to synthesize literature on your research topic is vital. Gardner (2008) admits that an effective synthesis is a considerable feat, but recommends four components to help achieve this: a goal, a starting point, a strategy/method, and written drafts with feedback.

For nurse researchers synthesizing previous research, this could entail an integrative review, narrative synthesis, meta-analysis, and metasynthesis. These last two methods of synthesizing literature are discussed in Chapter 3. Having a synthesizing mind is critical throughout a program of research, be it for a literature review, a grant proposal, or a manuscript to be submitted for publication.

With a creative mind, a person can break new ground and consider new ideas and ways of thinking. Creativity is especially important in qualitative research. Gardner (2008) warns us that creativity is never achieved by one individual or one small group, but instead depends on the interaction of three autonomous elements:

1. A person who has achieved mastery in a discipline or practice
2. The culture in which the person is working
3. The social field that surrounds the person

Key to a successful research program is collaboration within and across disciplines. Collaboration is discussed in Chapter 5 of this book. A respectful mind is needed to welcome and accept differences between persons and groups in order to understand others and to be able to work effectively with others.

Important for nursing, not only as a scholarly discipline but also as a clinical profession, is the ethical mind. As nurse researchers, our ethical conduct is most important. Our research aimed at addressing health care disparities and helping the most vulnerable populations depends on the ethical mind. Gardner (2008) describes this mind as one that "conceptualizes how workers can serve purposes beyond self-interest and how citizens can work unselfishly to improve the lot of all" (p. 3).

7 Summits

In his book 7 *Summits*, Hickey (2010), a nurse, shared his challenges and triumphs in achieving his goal of climbing the seven summits of the world. Each of these summits is the highest mountain on each of the seven continents of the world. Hickey strongly felt that it was the skill sets he learned in nursing that prepared him to achieve his quest for mountaineering. Hickey identified the "7 summits of life" that helped him achieve his goal and that can be used by anyone pursuing a goal, no matter what it is. These can be viewed as attributes that can help nurse researchers attain a successful research trajectory:

1. Balance in life
2. Physical wellness
3. Established goals
4. A positive attitude
5. Realization of one's potential
6. Yearning for success
7. The opportunity to create a legacy (Hickey, 2010, p. 20).

Although not specifically talking about a research program, Hickey (2010) has some excellent advice that nurse researchers can use when establishing goals. He says that each of us has an Everest in our life: a career goal, our finances, or our health, to name a few. Our quest to achieve our Everest involves our dreams, but there are also challenges that may hinder our success in reaching our summit. To help overcome these obstacles, Hickey suggests identifying short-, mid-, and long-term goals and setting dates and times for meeting these goals.

One entry in Hickey's My Everest blog follows. It caught my attention since he referred to the poem "The Road Not Taken":

> Robert Frost notes in the "The Road Not Taken" that taking the same path as everyone else will get you only average or mediocre results. To be unique, to contribute something new, you need to take a different course—your own. It is far easier to follow the beaten path and enjoy the security of conformity. The steps to

realizing your own potential begin first with a clear definition of your goals and objectives. (Hickey, 2010, p. 111)

Some other traits that successful nurse researchers need to have in their toolbox include, first, a passion for their topic of research. Only this passionate desire will help to continually motivate researchers along their path of inquiry and discovery. Persistence and motivation also go hand in hand in maintaining a sustained program of research. Other necessary personality traits are perseverance, dedication, tenacity, determination, and devotion.

Ideas for a Program of Research

How does someone get ideas for a program of research? Research ideas can come from a variety of sources: intellectual, personal, group, or worldview (Fiske, 2004). Existing perspectives from reviewing the literature may not adequately explain the phenomenon of interest. Contradictions in findings reported in published studies may be found and need to be further investigated. Published meta-analyses and meta-syntheses are gold mines for providing the big picture of the state of the science on a particular topic. Ideas can also come from external sources such as a funding agency's research priorities (Polit & Beck, 2012).

Fiske (2004) recommends a few principles that help to uncover a research idea to be studied: First, keep in mind the gaps in the knowledge base. Choose perspectives that are underrepresented, but without getting onto runaway bandwagons, as research in that area will be crowded and a new researcher will not stand out. It will be difficult to report anything new. Test out whether your research idea has general appeal. Fiske reminds scientists that "whatever you work on, follow your passion. Enjoy it. Study what intrigues you. Why else put up with all the grief associated with research?" (p. 76).

One of the best sources of ideas for a program of research can be your own clinical practice. I believe this is the most valuable and richest source for a clinical-based discipline, such as nursing. Are there immediate problems in your clinical area that need to be addressed? Is there a specific area in your clinical work that you are passionate about and where you have seen patterns or trends that need a research focus to help improve nursing care?

Perhaps you are drawn to a specific theory, nursing or borrowed, and you would like to study it to see if it can be used to predict patients' behaviors or outcomes of nursing interventions? Hypotheses can be deduced from this theory and tested.

Yet another source of research ideas can be found toward the end of published research studies where the authors suggest implications for future research. Here are a couple of examples from the end of two of my research articles on traumatic childbirth, where I make suggestions for ideas for future research studies. In my anniversary of birth trauma study (Beck, 2006b), I offered the following ideas for future research:

> Research has confirmed the negative effects that postpartum depression has on mother-infant interactions and on the children's cognitive and emotional development. Future research needs to focus on examining if birth trauma and PTSD due to childbirth have similar disruptions in maternal-child relationships. Also important to consider for future studies is the question of comorbidity with PTSD due to birth trauma. Research with PTSD not related to childbirth indicates that comorbid depression and other anxiety disorders are common. . . . Lastly, additional studies are needed to determine if women who do not have the outlet or ability to talk about their experiences as those in this study, who had access to the Internet and TABS [Trauma and Birth Stress], are different in their experiences regarding the anniversary of their traumatic births. (Beck, 2006b, p. 389)

At the end of the article where I published the findings of my study on posttraumatic stress disorder (PTSD) due to childbirth (Beck, 2004b), I made these suggestions for future research:

> Studies focusing on women who have gone on to have other children even after experiencing PTSD attributable to birth trauma are needed. A purposive study of women who had a healing experience with this subsequent labor and delivery could examine how this healing childbirth was different from the previous traumatic birth. Studies can be designed to evaluate the effectiveness of PTSD interventions using childbirth support groups or specific prevention strategies. (Beck, 2004b, p. 223)

A knowledge-driven focus is essential for generating ideas for a sustained program of research. Your clinical practice, theory, integrative reviews, funding agencies, and so on, can provide fruitful ideas for your next research study, but limiting yourself to one type of research method will detract from the potential value of your program of research for the discipline of nursing. Researchers need to be open-minded and flexible when deciding on the methods they use in their research trajectory.

Tables 2.1 and 2.2 present my ideas for conducting the studies in my research trajectory. Table 2.1 focuses on how I got my ideas for the studies in which I used quantitative methods, while Table 2.2 highlights my ideas for my qualitative methods studies. I will now provide a few examples of different sources of research ideas in my program of research on postpartum mood and anxiety disorders.

• TABLE 2.1 Ideas for Research Questions for Quantitative Research Studies

Quantitative Methods	Ideas for Research Questions
1. Postpartum depression: Its relation to maternity blues and length of stay (Beck, Reynolds, & Rutowski, 1992)	Hospital in Michigan had seed money and asked me to study which day in first week after birth mothers have most physical problems.
4. Postpartum depression checklist (Beck, 1995a)	Used results of my phenomenological study on postpartum depression (PPD) to develop checklist.
5. Effect of postpartum depression on maternal-infant interaction: A meta-analysis (Beck, 1995b)	With a view to designing intervention for PPD, did series of meta-analyses to know state of science to base intervention on.
8. Relationship between postpartum depression and infant temperament: A meta-analysis (Beck, 1996b)	
9. Predictors of postpartum depression: A meta-analysis (Beck, 1996c)	
10. Postpartum depression predictors inventory (Beck, 1998a)	Used findings from meta-analysis of predictors of PPD to develop inventory.
11. Effect of postpartum depression on child development: A meta-analysis (Beck, 1998b)	
13. Postpartum depression screening scale: development and psychometric properties (Beck & Gable, 2000; 2001a; 2001b)	Based on findings from my qualitative studies, it was time to develop a formal screening instrument.
16. Predictors of postpartum depression: an update (Beck, 2001)	Five years after first meta-analysis on predictors, I wanted to do another meta-analysis on the topic since a flurry of studies had been published.
19. Postpartum depression predictors inventory–revised (Beck, 2002c)	Revised PDPI based on findings from second meta-analysis of predictors of PPD.
21. Postpartum depression screening scale: Hispanic version (Beck & Gable, 2003; 2005)	Requests from clinicians for Postpartum Depression Screening Scale (PDSS) that could be used with Hispanic women.
27. Further development of the postpartum depression predictors inventory-revised (Beck, Records, & Rice, 2006)	Approached by nurse researcher with data from her study using PDSS.

(continued)

• TABLE 2.1 Ideas for Research Questions for Quantitative
Research Studies (*continued*)

Quantitative Methods	Ideas for Research Questions
28. PDSS telephone administration (Beck, 2007)	Requests by clinicians to use PDSS over the phone.
34. PTSD in new mothers: Results of a 2-stage U.S. national survey (Beck, Gable, Sakala, & Declercq, 2011a)	As a member of consulting team for Childbirth Connection's LTM II national survey, I had access to the data set.
35. PPD in new mothers: Results of a 2-stage U.S. national survey (Beck et al., 2011b)	
37. PDSS vs PHQ-9 in ethnically diverse sample (Beck, Kurz, & Gable, 2012)	Approached by researcher in social work with data on PDSS from her research.
38. PDSS—Hungarian version (Hegedus & Beck, 2012)	Approached by nurse researcher to translate PDSS into Hungarian.
40. Effects of DHA on postpartum depression (Judge, Beck, Durham, McKelvey, & Lammi-Keefe, 2014)	Approached by researcher in nutritional sciences to do a randomized control trial.

• TABLE 2.2 Ideas for Research Questions for Qualitative Research

Qualitative Methods	Ideas for Research Questions
2. Lived experience of postpartum depression: a phenomenological study (Beck, 1992)	Instrument used in first quantitative study on postpartum depression (PPD) only gave percent of women experiencing symptoms of PPD. No qualitative studies in literature were found that explored mothers' experiences.
3. Teetering on the edge: A substantive theory of postpartum depression (Beck, 1993)	Results of my phenomenological study of PPD focused on symptoms. Want to now investigate basic problem of PPD and process women use to resolve it.
4. Depressed mothers' nurses caring (Beck, 1995c)	Mothers in my qualitative studies painted negative picture of nurses' caring.
5. Postpartum depressed mothers' experiences interacting with their children (Beck, 1996a)	Results of my meta-analysis revealed large negative effect of PPD on mothers' interactions with their infants. I wanted mothers' experiences in their own words.

(*continued*)

• TABLE 2.2 Ideas for Research Questions for Qualitative Research (*continued*)

Qualitative Methods	Ideas for Research Questions
12. Postpartum onset of panic disorder: A phenomenological study (Beck, 1998c)	Some mothers in my qualitative studies reported being given incorrect diagnoses of PPD when they really had panic disorder. Need to differentiate experiences.
17. Releasing the pause button: Grounded theory of first year of life of mothers of multiples (Beck, 2002a)	Findings from my study testing psychometrics of my Postpartum Depression Screening Scale (PDSS) indicated a high percentage of women who had given birth to twins had PPD. I wanted to get in-depth picture of what twin life was like.
18. Mothering multiples: A metasynthesis (Beck, 2002b)	At this time, metasynthesis was gaining momentum, and I wanted to synthesize research on mothering multiples.
20. Postpartum depression: A metasynthesis (Beck, 2002d)	Qualitative studies on PPD were accumulating in the literature, and I decided to synthesize them.
22. Birth trauma: In the eye of the beholder (Beck, 2004a)	At conference in New Zealand, met executive director of Trauma and Birth Stress (TABS), and we discussed my conducting research with mothers in TABS. Started series of studies.
23. PTSD after childbirth (Beck, 2004b)	
25. Pentadic cartography: Mapping birth trauma narratives (Beck, 2006a)	Had 11 additional narratives from my phenomenological study on birth trauma, and wanted to use different qualitative design.
26. Anniversary of birth trauma (Beck, 2006b)	A quote from a mother in a previous study on PTSD gave me the idea.
29. First grounded theory modification (Beck, 2007)	Invited to write a chapter updating my Teetering on the Edge grounded theory of PPD.
30. Impact of birth trauma on breastfeeding (Beck & Watson, 2008)	
31. Adult survivor of child abuse and her breastfeeding experience: A case study (Beck, 2009a)	One mother in study on impact of birth trauma on breastfeeding shared in-depth narrative of impact of her child sexual abuse.

(*continued*)

• TABLE 2.2 Ideas for Research Questions for Qualitative Research (*continued*)

Qualitative Methods	Ideas for Research Questions
32. The arm: No escaping reality for mothers of children with OBPI (Beck, 2009b)	Some of the mothers in my qualitative studies had infants with obstetric brachial plexus injuries (OBPI) as result of traumatic births. They were members of United Brachial Plexus Network (UBPN), and I was invited to speak at their conference.
33. Subsequent childbirth after a previous traumatic birth (Beck & Watson, 2010)	
36. Meta-ethnography of traumatic childbirth (Beck, 2011)	After conducting six studies on birth trauma, it was time to synthesize my research findings.
39. Second grounded theory modification (Beck, 2012)	Second modification of my Teetering on the Edge grounded theory for new edition of textbook chapter.
38. Secondary traumatic stress of OB nurses (Beck & Gable, 2012)	When I presented my birth trauma research at conferences, labor and delivery nurses would often say I needed to study them. Nurses were as traumatized as the mothers.
42. Fathers' experiences of witnessing their partners' traumatic childbirth (Beck et al., 2013)	Mothers in previous studies on birth trauma would often say, "You should study my husband; he was as traumatized as I was."
43. Mothers' experiences of EMDR therapy (Beck et al., 2013)	Mothers would email me asking what this type of therapy was like.
44. Obstetric nightmare of shoulder dystocia (Beck, 2013)	Decided to do qualitative secondary analysis of data from earlier qualitative studies.
45. Secondary traumatic stress in CNMs (Beck, LoGiudice, & Gable, 2015)	At conference where I spoke of secondary traumatic stress (STS) in L&D nurses, certified nurse midwives (CNMs) would say I needed to study them too.
In Progress	
46. Post-traumatic growth after traumatic childbirth.	In the literature, researchers have reported posttraumatic growth in trauma victims. No research had been done yet with traumatic childibirth.

Serendipitous

Sometimes, a research idea for a study is serendipitous. At one point in my research program I was fortunate enough to be at the right place at the right time. The year was 2000, and I was delivering the keynote address at the Australasian Marcé International Society's conference in Christchurch, New Zealand. The conference organizers had asked me to focus on my phenomenological study of postpartum-onset panic disorder but to also describe the range of anxiety disorders women can experience both in pregnancy and in the postpartum period. In preparing for this keynote, I came across a handful of quantitative studies published on posttraumatic stress disorder (PTSD) due to childbirth. I had not heard of this postpartum anxiety disorder before reading these few studies. I did briefly mention PTSD due to childbirth in my keynote. Later at the conference, a mother who had suffered with PTSD due to a traumatic birth vividly shared her personal experience. This mother, Sue Watson, had started a charitable trust in New Zealand, called Trauma and Birth Stress (TABS), that provides support to mothers who have experienced birth trauma (www.tabs.org.nz). During lunch, I spoke with this mother regarding the possibility of conducting some qualitative research with the mothers in TABS. That chance meeting at the conference that day in 2000 was the start of over a decade of my research on traumatic childbirth and its resulting PTSD.

Qualitative Research

If your research program involves qualitative research, quotes of participants in your earlier studies can produce some of the best ideas for what to study next. I will illustrate this point with two examples from my studies. To date, I have conducted a series of eight qualitative studies on traumatic childbirth. The second study in this series was entitled "Post-traumatic stress disorder due to childbirth: The aftermath" (Beck, 2004b). In the data from that study I got the idea to conduct two other qualitative studies regarding the chronic effects of traumatic birth. One mother who had experienced a severe postpartum hemorrhage 3 years earlier provided a glimpse into the struggles when the anniversary of her birth trauma occurred, which was also her child's birthday:

> My child turned 3 years old a few weeks ago. I suppose the pain was not so acute this time. I actually made him a birthday cake and was grateful that I could go to work and not think about the significance of the day. The pain was less, but it was replaced by a numbness that still worries me. I hope that as time passes I can forge some kind of real closeness with this child. I am still unable to tell him I love him, but I can now hold him and have times when I am proud of him. I have come a long, long way. (Beck, 2004b, p. 222)

Because of this powerful quote, I got the idea to conduct a phenomenological study in 2006 titled, "The anniversary of birth trauma: Failure to rescue" (Beck, 2006b). In that study, "Four themes revealed the meaning of

women's experiences of the anniversary of their birth trauma: (a) The prologue: An agonizing time; (b) The actual day: A celebration of a birthday or
the torment of an anniversary; (c) The epilogue: A fragile state; and (d) Subsequent anniversaries: For better or worse" (Beck, 2006b, p. 381).

Another quote from my 2004b study on PTSD after a traumatic birth
gave me another idea for a study, this time on subsequent childbirth following a previous birth trauma (Beck & Watson, 2010). This telling quote was as
follows:

> I couldn't envision *ever* having another baby. There was no way
> I could expose myself again to that degree of vulnerability and
> abandonment. My little girl was the most precious thing in my
> life, but events that occurred at the birth mean that I will not be
> having any more children. I had a tubal ligation, and I grieved for
> the babies I thought I wouldn't have. (Beck, 2004a, p. 222)

In this phenomenological study of subsequent childbirth following birth
trauma with 35 mothers from around the globe, four themes emerged: "(a) Rid-
ing the turbulent wave of panic during pregnancy; (b) Strategizing: Attempts
to reclaim their body and complete the journey to motherhood; (c) Bringing
reverence to the birthing process and empowering women; and (d) Still elu-
sive: The longed-for healing birth experience" (Beck & Watson, 2010, p. 241).

Unused Data

Sometimes in your program of research, you may have extra data you do
not need for the study you are currently analyzing. Do not just put those
unused data away in a file cabinet. Think of a way you can conduct another
study using those data. This happened to me in my research program. I
had been conducting my first study on traumatic childbirth (Beck, 2004a).
It was a phenomenological study where mothers from around the globe
sent me their stories of their birth trauma. I had finished analyzing stories
from 40 mothers and had achieved data saturation long before I had got-
ten to the 40th mother. Once I completed data analysis, 11 more mothers
participated in this Internet study. I still had my Institutional Review Board
(IRB) protocol open, and so I set out to use these additional 11 stories using
a different qualitative research design. Which design, though, was the question. I knew another phenomenological study was not necessary since I had
achieved data saturation well before I had covered 40 participants. After
reviewing different qualitative research designs, I decided on narrative inquiry. I then had to decide what type of narrative analysis approach would
best fit the birth trauma narratives. I read the primary sources of these

different approaches and chose Burke's (1969) dramatistic pentad to provide the structure for this narrative analysis. Burke's analysis uses five key elements of a story: act, scene, agent, agency, and purpose; rather, These five components are not meant to be understood as individual elements; rather, these elements are paired together as ratios such as scene:agent. An imbalance between ratios is what is looked for; that is, the tension between ratios. Act:agency was the problematic ratio that appeared most often in traumatic childbirth. It was how an act to a mother was done in such an uncaring manner that it was problematic. Table 2.3 presents the ratio imbalances in the 11 mothers' birth trauma narratives (Beck, 2006a). The ratio imbalances from

• TABLE 2.3 Ratio Imbalances in Mothers' Birth Trauma Stories

	Birth Trauma	Scene	Ratio Imbalance
1	On the postpartum unit delivery of a nonliving preterm infant	Scene 1	Scene:Agent
		Scene 2	Act:Agency
		Scene 3	Act:Agency
2	Emergency cesarean of a preterm infant due to mother's hemorrhaging; infant to neonatal intensive care unit	Scene 1	Act:Agency
		Scene 2	Scene:Agent
3	Emergency cesarean due to "baby being stuck"	Scene 1	Act:Agent
4	Hemorrhaging due to vasa previa; emergency cesarean	Scene 1	Act:Agency
		Scene 2	Act:Agent
5	Multiple insertions for epidural; mother's blood pressure dropped; fetal heart rate dropped, leading to a crisis	Scene 1	Act:Agency
		Scene 2	Act:Agency
6	Mother sustained nerve damage due to two forceps deliveries of her twins; her left foot and leg paralyzed	Scene 1	Scene:Agent
		Scene 2	Act:Agency
		Scene 3	Act:Agency
		Scene 4	Agent:Act
7	Postpartum hemorrhage after water birth	Scene 1	Scene:Agent
8	Epidural did not work, but labor and delivery (L&D) staff did not believe mother; forceps delivery without pain medication	Scene 1	Act:Agency

(continued)

• TABLE 2.3 Ratio Imbalances in Mothers' Birth Trauma Stories (*continued*)

	Birth Trauma	Scene	Ratio Imbalance
9	Mother in active labor, but L&D staff did not believe her; vacuum extraction without any pain medication; mother hemorrhaged	Scene 1	Act : Agency
		Scene 2	Act : Agency
10	Mother induced against her wishes; first twin delivered vaginally; second twin delivered by cesarean	Scene 1	Act : Agency
		Scene 2	Act : Agency
		Scene 3	Act : Agency
11	Mother's pelvis dislocated when nurse yanked bedpan away	Scene 1	Act : Agency
		Scene 2	Act : Agency

Reprinted with permission from Beck (2006a, p. 459).

my narrative analysis confirmed the themes that emerged in my earlier phenomenological study of birth trauma (Beck, 2004a). Keeping women's stories as a whole in narrative analysis, however, allowed the sequencing of events in each traumatic birth. It revealed the multiple traumatic insults these mothers suffered during their labor and delivery that were not apparent in the phenomenological study.

"You Ought to Study Us"

My idea for my mixed methods study came about in the following way. As I was presenting papers at conferences on my traumatic childbirth research, often someone in the audience who happened to be a labor and delivery nurse would say, "You ought to research us. We are as traumatized as the mothers are!" How grateful I am to these nurses for offering their insightful suggestions to me for my program of research. Without their comments, I would never have even thought to follow this path. So after repeatedly hearing this plea, I reviewed the literature and discovered "secondary traumatic stress." Figley (1995) defined this as stress clinicians can experience that "results from helping or wanting to help a traumatized or suffering person" (p. 10). It is an occupational hazard for clinicians who care for patients who are traumatized. Secondary traumatic stress is a syndrome of symptoms similar to PTSD. This syndrome had been reported in the literature in oncology, emergency department, heart and vascular, forensic, pediatric, and hospice nurses. However, no research had been conducted to examine secondary traumatic stress in labor and delivery nurses. This discovery led me on, in my program of re-search, down the mixed methods path. Since no research, either quantitative or qualitative, had yet been done on this topic, I not only wanted to learn about labor and delivery nurses' experiences of attending traumatic births but also felt it was important to quantitatively get a handle on the prevalence of secondary traumatic stress in this specialty of nursing. "Therefore, the pur-poses of this mixed methods study were to (a) determine the prevalence and severity of secondary traumatic stress in L&D nurses by obtaining quantita-tive data from a survey of L&D nurses using the Secondary Traumatic Stress Scale (STSS; Bride, Robinson, Yegidis, & Figley, 2004) and (b) explore those results in more depth through content analysis of the nurses' descriptions of their experiences attending traumatic births" (Beck & Gable, 2012, p. 748).

Using a convergent parallel design for mixed methods research from data in the quantitative strand, we found that 35% of the sample of labor and delivery nurses reported moderate to severe levels of secondary traumatic stress. Also, 26% of the sample met all the *Diagnostic and Statistical Manual of Mental Disorders,* fourth edition *(DSM-IV)* diagnostic criteria for screen-ing positive for PTSD due to exposure to their laboring patients who were traumatized. Focusing on the data from the qualitative strand of this mixed methods study, content analysis of the nurses' descriptions of being pres-ent at traumatic births revealed six themes: (a) magnifying the exposure to traumatic births, (b) struggling to maintain a professional role while with traumatized patients, (c) agonizing over what should have been, (d) mitigat-ing the aftermath of exposure to traumatic births, (e) haunted by secondary traumatic stress symptoms, and (f) considering forgoing careers in labor and delivery to survive (Beck & Gable, 2012).

Other Nurse Researchers' Sources of Research Ideas

Having provided examples of sources of ideas for research studies from my own research trajectory, I shall now present a few from other nurse researchers.

Judith Wuest

Using feminist grounded theory methods, Wuest (1998, 2001) developed a mid-range theory of precarious ordering for Canadian women who were caring for family members with acute and chronic illnesses. Wuest discovered that ap-proximately 15% of the women in her research were providing care to family members who had previously abused them. The course of Wuest's research pro-gram then took a serendipitous turn from qualitative to quantitative research.

As Wuest et al. (2006) explained, this next study "began with an un-likely alliance between Wuest, a grounded theorist, and Hodgins who views the world through a quantitative lens" (p. 26). Wuest did not know, but Hodgins had nursing students in her course critique Wuest's grounded theory study (1998). Following this class, Wuest and Hodgins met in the hallway, and Hodgins expressed her view that Wuest's theory of precarious ordering presented some hypotheses that called for some quantitative studies and testing. At first Wuest argued against the use of quantitative methods to further her grounded theory. As she continued her research, Wuest realized that her extension of her theory using qualitative methods would not yield the necessary data regarding the prevalence of the health problem or scope of health effects that was essential for policy decisions. Her chance meeting in the hallway with Hodgins led Wuest to approach Hodgins to form a research team to develop an instrument derived from her grounded theory. Hodgins took the lead in the instrument development of the Caregiving Survey, while Wuest contributed to the conceptual understanding from the grounded theory (Wuest & Hodgins, 2011).

Ruth McCorkle

Her purposeful research path toward making a difference in cancer care was guided by a major turning point in her life when she volunteered for the U.S. Air Force Corps during the Vietnam War. Caring for critically wounded soldiers who often died from battle wounds taught McCorkle how to be present with these young men and their families as they faced death. After completing her military service, McCorkle obtained her master's and doctoral degrees to provide the foundation she would need to develop and test the effects of clinical interventions on improving nursing care to patients with cancer and their families. As McCorkle shared:

> A diagnosis of cancer still evokes fear and anxiety and patients question whether their lives will end prematurely and in pain. These primordial emotions have been the core of my research, to make their diagnosis and treatment bearable so they can go on with living their lives the best they can. I have used the rigor of science to hone in on what nurses do to preserve the humanness of patients and families in cancer care. The essence of what we do is to form a relationship with patients during that raw experience of vulnerability to guide them through their cancer journey. This is what my experience in Vietnam taught me; it was my presence that mattered to the young soldiers and their family members. (McCorkle, 2011, p. 339)

Karin Olson

Olson (2013) shared that her interest in researching fatigue peaked when she was the coordinator of nursing research in Canada at a large cancer center.

A nurse in the outpatient clinic told Olson about a patient who had withdrawn from a curative protocol for his colorectal cancer because he was "too tired" and he could not cope with his unbearable lack of energy. Olson decided that her next path would be to do some observation in the outpatient clinic to meet with patients with fatigue. To her surprise, although the majority of patients experienced fatigue, some persons with advanced cancer who were undergoing aggressive treatment did not state they were fatigued. Olson questioned whether these patients were denying their fatigue, whether for some reason they did not want to admit they were fatigued, or whether they were really not fatigued, and if not, why not.

These unanswered questions led Olson to decide to explore fatigue through her research. She wanted to understand why some patients reported being fatigued, while other patients with the same cancer treatment protocol did not. After reviewing the literature and finding a lack of research on the absence of fatigue in those patients who would be expected to experience significant fatigue, Olson started her research program on fatigue with a qualitative study, specifically grounded theory. Out of all the qualitative designs Olson could have used, she chose grounded theory because her earlier observations in the outpatient clinic revealed that social interactions greatly impacted the manner in which patients experienced their cancer treatment. Since grounded theory is rooted in symbolic interaction and focuses on social processes, Olson saw it as the most appropriate qualitative path to answer her research questions.

Janice Morse

Morse explained how she began her research program on suffering.

> I came to the study of suffering theory by the back door, so to speak. My primary interest is in comfort (Morse, 1992) and it took me several years to understand that to fully comprehend the nature of comfort and comforting I had to first understand what was being comforted (Morse, 1999). I needed to explore the nature of patient discomfort, to learn about patient cues and signals of distress, and, in general, how discomforts were endured, experienced, eased, and relieved. (Morse, 2002, p. 118)

REFERENCES

Beck, C. T. (1992). The lived experience of postpartum depression: A phenomenological study. *Nursing Research, 41*, 166–170.

Beck, C. T. (1993). Qualitative research: The evaluation of its credibility, fittingness and auditability. *Western Journal of Nursing Research, 15*, 263–266.

Beck, C. T. (1995a). Screening methods for postpartum depression. *Journal of Obstetric, Gynecologic, and Neonatal Nursing, 24*, 308–312.

Beck, C. T. (1995b). The effect of postpartum depression of maternal-infant interaction: A meta-analysis. *Nursing Research, 44,* 298–304.

Beck, C. T. (1995c). Perceptions of nurses' caring by mothers experiencing postpartum depression. *Journal of Obstetric, Gynecologic, and Neonatal Nursing, 24,* 819–825.

Beck, C. T. (1996a). Postpartum depressed mothers' experiences interacting with their children. *Nursing Research, 45* (2), 98–104.

Beck, C. T. (1996b). The relationship between postpartum depression and infant temperament: A meta-analysis. *Nursing Research, 45,* 225–230.

Beck, C. T. (1996c). Predictors of postpartum depression: A meta-analysis. *Nursing Research, 45,* 297–303.

Beck, C. T. (1998a). A checklist to identify women at risk for developing postpartum depression. *Journal of Obstetric, Gynecologic, and Neonatal Nursing, 27,* 39–46.

Beck, C. T. (1998b). Effects of postpartum depression on child development: A meta-analysis. *Archives of Psychiatric Nursing, 12,* 12–20.

Beck, C. T. (1998c). Postpartum onset of panic disorder. *Image: Journal of Nursing Scholarship, 30,* 131–135.

Beck, C. T. (2001). Predictors of postpartum depression: An update. *Nursing Research, 50,* 275–285.

Beck, C. T. (2002a). Releasing the pause button: Mothering twins during the first year of life. *Qualitative Health Research, 12,* 593–608.

Beck, C. T. (2002b). Mothering multiples: A meta-synthesis of the qualitative research. *MCN: The American Journal of Maternal Child Nursing, 27,* 214–221.

Beck, C. T. (2002c). Revision of the postpartum depression predictors inventory. *Journal of the Obstetric, Gynecologic, and Neonatal Nursing, 31,* 394–402.

Beck, C. T. (2002d). Postpartum depression: A meta-synthesis of qualitative research. *Qualitative Health Research, 12,* 453–472.

Beck, C. T. (2004a). Birth trauma: In the eye of the beholder, *Nursing Research, 53*(1), 28–35.

Beck, C. T. (2004b). Post-traumatic stress disorder due to childbirth: The aftermath, *Nursing Research, 53*(4), 216–224.

Beck, C. T. (2006a). Pentadic cartography: Mapping birth trauma narratives. *Qualitative Health Research, 16* (4), 453–466.

Beck, C. T. (2006b). The anniversary of birth trauma: Failure to rescue. *Nursing Research, 55,* 381–390.

Beck, C. T. (2007). Exemplar: Teetering on the edge: A continually emerging theory of postpartum depression. In P. L. Munhall (ed.), *Nursing research: A qualitative perspective* (4th ed., pp. 273–292). Sudbury, MA: Jones & Bartlett.

Beck, C. T. (2009a). An adult survivor of childhood sexual abuse and her breastfeeding experience: A case study. *MCN: American Journal of Maternal Child Nursing, 34,* 91–97.

Beck, C. T. (2009b). The arm: There's no escaping the reality for mothers caring for their children with obstetric brachial plexus injuries. *Nursing Research, 58,* 237–45.

Beck, C. T. (2011). A metaethnography of traumatic childbirth and its aftermath: Amplifying causal looping. *Qualitative Health Research, 21,* 301–311.

Beck, C. T. (2012). Exemplar: Teetering on the edge: A second grounded theory modification. In P. L. Munhall (ed.), *Nursing research: A qualitative perspective* (5th ed., pp. 257–284) Sudbury, MA: Jones & Bartlett.

Beck, C. T. (2013). The obstetric nightmare of shoulder dystocia: A tale from two perspectives. *MCN: The American Journal of Maternal Child Nursing, 38,* 34–40.

Beck, C. T., Driscoll, J. W., & Watson, S. (2013). *Traumatic childbirth.* New York, NY: Routledge Publishers.

Beck, C. T., & Gable, R. K. (2000). Postpartum Depression Screening Scale: Development and psychometric testing. *Nursing Research, 49,* 272-282.

Beck, C. T., & Gable, R. K. (2003). Postpartum Depression Screening Scale—Spanish version. *Nursing Research, 52,* 296–306.

Beck, C. T., & Gable, R. K. (2012). Secondary traumatic stress in labor and delivery nurses: A mixed methods study. *Journal of Obstetric, Gynecologic, and Neonatal Nursing, 41,* 747–760.

Beck, C. T., Gable, R. K., Sakala, C., & Declercq, E. R. (2011a). Posttraumatic stress disorder in new mothers: Results from a two-stage U.S. national survey. *Birth, 38,* 216–227.

Beck, C. T., Gable, R. K., Sakala, C., & Declercq, E. R. (2011b). Postpartum depression in new mothers: Results from a two-stage U.S. national survey. *Journal of Midwifery and Women's Health, 56,* 427–435.

Beck, C. T., Kurz, B., & Gable, R. K. (2012). Concordance and discordance of the Postpartum Depression Screening Scale (PDSS) and the Patient Health Questionnaire-9 (PHQ-9) in an ethnically diverse sample. *Journal of Social Service Research, 38,* 439–450.

Beck, C.T., LoGiudice, J., & Gable, R.K. (2015). Shaken belief in the birth process: A mixed methods study of secondary traumatic stress in certified nurse-midwives. *Journal of Midwifery & Women's Health, 60,* 16-23.

Beck, C. T., Records, K., & Rice, M. (2006). Further validation of the Postpartum Depression Predictors Inventory-Revised. *Journal of Obstetric, Gynecologic, and Neonatal Nursing, 35,* 735–745.

Beck, C. T., Reynolds, M., & Rutowski, P. (1992). Maternity blues and postpartum depression. *Journal of Obstetric, Gynecologic, and Neonatal Nursing, 21,* 287–293.

Beck, C. T., & Watson, S. (2008). The impact of birth trauma on breastfeeding: A tale of two pathways. *Nursing Research, 57,* 228–236.

Beck, C. T., & Watson, S. (2010). Subsequent childbirth after a previous traumatic birth. *Nursing Research, 59,* 241–249.

Bride, B. E., Robinson, M. M., Yegidis, B., & Figley, C. R. (2004). Development and validation of the Secondary Traumatic Stress Scale. *Research on Social Work Practice, 14,* 27–35.

Burke, K. (1969). *A grammar of motives.* Berkley, CA: University of California Press.

Conn, V. S. (2004). Building a research trajectory. *Western Journal of Nursing Research, 26*(6), 592–594.

Figley, C. R. (1995). Compassion fatigue: Toward a new understanding of the costs of caring. In B. H. Stamm (ed.), *Secondary traumatic stress: Self-care issues for clinicians, researchers, and educators* (pp. 3–28). Lutherville, MD: Sidran Press.

Fiske, S. T. (2004). Developing a program of research. In C. Sansone, C. C. Mork, & A. T. Panter (Eds.), *The SAGE handbook of methods in social psychology* (pp. 71–90). Thousand Oaks, CA: SAGE.

Gardner, H. (2008). *5 Minds for the future.* Boston, MA: Harvard Business Press.

Hegedus, K., & Beck, C. T. (2012). Development and psychometric testing of the Post-partum Depression Screening Scale: Hungarian version. *International Journal for Human Caring, 16,* 54–58.

Hickey, P. (2010). *7 Summits: A nurse's quest to conquer mountaineering and life.* Sudbury, MA: Jones & Bartlett.

Judge, M. P., Beck, C. T., Durham, H., McKelvey, M. M., & Lammi-Keefe, C. (2014) Pilot trial evaluating maternal DHA consumption during pregnancy decreases postpartum depressive symptomatology. *International Journal of Nursing Sciences, 1,* 339–345.

Kroeker, G. (2008). Forest paths metaphor. Retrieved from www.garthkroeker .blogspot.com

McCorkle, R. (2011). A purposeful career path to make a difference in cancer care. *Cancer Nursing, 34*(4), 335–339.

Morse, J. M. (1992). Comfort: The refocusing of nursing care. *Clinical Nursing Research, 1,* 91–113.

Morse, J. M. (1999). Qualitative methods: The state of the art. *Qualitative Health Research, 9*(3), 393–406.

Morse, J. M. (2002). Qualitative health research: Challenges for the 21st century. *Qualitative Health Research, 12*(1), 116–129.

Morse, J. M. (2005). Qualitative research is not a modification of quantitative research. *Qualitative Health Research, 15,* 1003–1005.

Morse, J. M. (2010). What happened to research programs? *Qualitative Health Research, 20*(2), 147.

Olson, K. (2013). Learning about the nature of fatigue. In C. T. Beck (Ed.), *Routledge international handbook of qualitative nursing research* (pp. 64–74). New York, NY: Routledge.

Polit, D. F., & Beck, C. T. (2012). *Nursing research: Generating and assessing evidence for nursing practice.* Philadelphia, PA: Wolters Kluwer Health/Lippincott Williams & Wilkins.

White, H. (1998). *Paths and walkways: Simple projects, contemporary designs.* San Francisco, CA: Chronicle Books.

Wuest, J. (1998). Setting boundaries: A strategy for precarious ordering of women's caring demands. *Research in Nursing & Health, 21,* 39–49.

Wuest, J. (2001). Precarious ordering: Toward a formal theory of women's caring [Special volume. Using grounded theory in study of women's health]. *Health Care for Women International, 22,* 1–2, 167–193.

Wuest, J., & Hodgins, M. J. (2011). Reflections on methodological approaches and conceptual contributions on a program of caregiving research: Development and testing of Wuest's theory of family caregiving. *Qualitative Health Research, 21*(2), 151–161.

Wuest, J., Hodgins, M. J., Merritt-Gray, M., Seaman, P., Malcolm, J., & Furlong, K. (2006). Queries and quandaries in developing and testing an instrument derived from a grounded theory. *The Journal of Theory Construction and Testing, 10*(1), 26–33.

T·H·R·E·E

Planning Sequential Studies

We must choose each step we take with utmost caution,
for the footprints we leave behind are as important
as the path we will follow.
—*Lori R. Lopez, Dance of the Chupacabras*

As noted in the second chapter, the backbone of my perspective in developing a valuable research program for a discipline, such as nursing, is that it be knowledge driven and not method limited. The sequence of studies in a research trajectory is not fixed ahead of time. When starting a research trajectory, a researcher cannot predict what paths that program will take and the direction in which subsequent research studies will lead the researcher. It is only after the completion of one study that a researcher can decide the most appropriate step to be taken next. Whether the next study should be qualitative, quantitative, or mixed methods and what specific research design needs to be used should be based on the results of the previous study in the research trajectory and also on the current state of knowledge in this substantive area. At each juncture, the progression of a program of research can take many different paths.

Tables 3.1 and 3.2 illustrate the different paths my research program took as it turned from a quantitative to a qualitative study and back again. These changes in the direction of my path in using either quantitative, qualitative, or mixed methods designs were dictated by the results of my previous studies. For the purpose of these tables, I have listed one study after another, but many times in my research trajectory I conducted multiple studies simultaneously. Through the description of my research program on postpartum mood and anxiety disorders, I also hope to illustrate how my qualitative studies put the flesh on the bones of my quantitative studies and added the tears to the statistics. The path my research trajectory has taken

• **TABLE 3.1 Postpartum Mood and Anxiety Disorders Research Program**

Quantitative Methods	Qualitative Methods
1. Postpartum depression: Its relation to maternity blues and length of stay (Beck et al., 1992)	
	2. Lived experience of postpartum depression: A phenomenological study (Beck, 1992)
	3. Teetering on the edge: A substantive theory of postpartum depression (Beck, 1993)
4. Postpartum depression checklist (Beck, 1995a)	
5. Effect of postpartum depression on maternal-infant interaction: A meta-analysis (Beck, 1995b)	
	6. Depressed mothers' nurses caring (Beck, 1995c)
	7. Postpartum depressed mothers' experiences interacting with their children (Beck, 1996a)
8. Relationship between postpartum depression and infant temperament: A meta-analysis (Beck, 1996b)	
9. Predictors of postpartum depression: A meta-analysis (Beck, 1996c)	
10. Postpartum depression predictors inventory (Beck, 1998a)	
11. Effect of postpartum depression on child development: A meta-analysis (Beck, 1998b)	
	12. Postpartum onset of panic disorder: A phenomenological study (Beck, 1998c)
13. Postpartum depression screening scale: Development and psychometric properties (Beck & Gable, 2000)	

(continued)

• TABLE 3.1 Postpartum Mood and Anxiety Disorders
Research Program (*continued*)

Quantitative Methods	Qualitative Methods
14. Further validation of the PDSS (Beck & Gable, 2001a)	
15. Comparative analysis of three depression screening scales (Beck & Gable, 2001b)	
16. Predictors of postpartum depression: An update (Beck, 2001)	
	17. Releasing the pause button: Grounded theory of first year of life of mothers of multiples (Beck, 2002a)
	18. Mothering multiples: A metasynthesis (Beck, 2002b)
19. Postpartum depression predictors inventory—revised (Beck, 2002c)	
	20. Postpartum depression: A metasynthesis (Beck, 2002d)
21. Postpartum Depression Screening Scale: Spanish version (Beck & Gable, 2003)	
	22. Birth trauma: In the eye of the beholder (Beck, 2004a)
	23. PTSD after childbirth (Beck, 2004b)
24. Screening performance of PDSS-spanish version (Beck & Gable, 2005)	
	25. Pentadic cartography: mapping birth trauma narratives (Beck, 2006a)
	26. Anniversary of birth trauma (Beck, 2006b)
27. Further development of the postpartum depression predictors inventory—revised (Beck et al., 2006)	
28. PDSS telephone administration (Beck, 2007)	

(*continued*)

• **TABLE 3.1 Postpartum Mood and Anxiety Disorders Research Program** (*continued*)

Quantitative Methods	Qualitative Methods
	29. First grounded theory modification (Beck, 2007)
	30. Impact of birth trauma on breastfeeding (Beck & Watson, 2008)
	31. Adult survivor of child abuse and her breastfeeding experience: A case study (Beck, 2009a)
	32. The arm: No escaping reality for mothers of children with OBPI (Beck, 2009b)
	33. Subsequent childbirth after a previous traumatic birth (Beck & Watson, 2010)
34. PTSD in new mothers: Results of a 2-stage US national survey (Beck et al., 2011a)	
35. PPD in new mothers: Results of a 2-stage US national survey (Beck et al., 2011b)	
	36. Meta-ethnography of traumatic childbirth (Beck, 2011)
37. PDSS vs. PHQ-9 in ethnically diverse sample (Beck, Kurz, & Gable 2012)	
38. PDSS-hungarian version (Hegedus & Beck, 2012)	
	39. Second grounded theory modification (Beck, 2012)
40. Effects of DHA on postpartum depression (Judge et al., 2014)	
41. Secondary traumatic stress of OB nurses (Beck, 2012)	
	42. Fathers' experiences of witnessing their partners' traumatic childbirth (Beck et al., 2013)

(*continued*)

• **TABLE 3.1 Postpartum Mood and Anxiety Disorders Research Program (*continued*)**

Quantitative Methods	Qualitative Methods
	43. Mothers' experiences of EMDR therapy (Beck et al., 2013)
	44. Obstetric nightmare of shoulder dystocia (Beck, 2013)
45. Secondary traumatic stress in CNMs (Beck et al., 2015)	
In Progress	
	46. Post traumatic growth after traumatic Childbirth

• **TABLE 3.2 Sequential Pathways in Postpartum Mood and Anxiety Research Program**

Study Numbers	Sequential Pathways
1–3	Quantitative – Qualitative – Qualitative
4–6	Quantitative – Quantitative – Qualitative
7–9	Qualitative – Quantitative – Quantitative
10–12	Quantitative – Quantitative – Qualitative
13–15	Quantitative – Quantitative – Quantitative
16–18	Quantitative – Qualitative – Qualitative
19–21	Quantitative – Qualitative – Quantitative
22–24	Qualitative – Qualitative – Quantitative
25–27	Qualitative – Qualitative – Quantitative
28–30	Quantitative – Qualitative – Qualitative
31–33	Qualitative – Qualitative – Qualitative
34–36	Quantitative – Quantitative – Qualitative
37–39	Quantitative – Quantitative – Qualitative
40–42	Quantitative – Mixed Methods – Qualitative
43–45	Qualitative – Qualitative – Mixed Methods
46	Qualitative

over the years is something I could never have mapped out ahead of time. I had no idea, for example, that one phase of my research trajectory would involve instrument development of the Postpartum Depression Screening Scale (Beck & Gable, 2002).

THE LONG AND WINDING PATH OF THE RESEARCH PROGRAM ON POSTPARTUM MOOD AND ANXIETY DISORDERS

In my first study, I quantitatively investigated the relationship between maternity blues and postpartum depression (Beck, Reynolds, & Rutowski, 1992). In addition, I compared the levels of postpartum depressive symptoms in two groups of new mothers: traditional stay versus early discharge from the hospital. Mothers in this study were followed from birth through the first 3 months postpartum. Women completed the Beck Depression Inventory (BDI; Beck, Ward, Mendelson, Mock, & Erbaugh, 1961). Once this first study was completed, I searched the literature, which did not reveal any qualitative studies on postpartum depression. What I wanted to study next was what mothers with postpartum depression were experiencing in their own words. So the second study in my program of research was a qualitative one, specifically, a phenomenological study focusing on the research question "What is the meaning of women's experiences of postpartum depression?" Findings of this study revealed 11 themes that powerfully described the essence of the experience of postpartum depression (Beck, 1992).

For my third study, I again chose to stay with qualitative methods. My purpose was to learn more about postpartum depression from the mothers' perspective. The research questions that now needed to be answered were "What is the basic social psychological problem mothers with postpartum depression experience?" and "What is the social psychological process mothers use to cope with and resolve postpartum depression?" These research questions could only be answered by a grounded theory study, which is the path I took (Beck, 1993). Data analysis revealed that loss of control was the basic problem and women resolved this problem by a four-stage process called teetering on the edge.

In both of the qualitative studies I had just completed, women briefly shared the difficulties they had experienced interacting with their infants while in the depths of their postpartum depression. At this choice of a path in my research trajectory, I made the decision to further examine this particular aspect of postpartum depression. In my literature review, I located 19 quantitative studies that had been conducted on the effect of postpartum depression on mother–infant interaction. To determine just how large an effect postpartum depression had on mother–infant interaction, I conducted a meta-analysis of those 19 quantitative studies (Beck, 1995b). So, at these crossroads in my research program, I crossed back over to quantitative methods. The meta-analysis revealed a large adverse effect size of postpartum depression on maternal–infant interaction during the first year of life. On completing this meta-analysis, I went back to the literature to see if there were any published qualitative studies to put the "flesh on the bones" of this quantitative effect size revealed in my meta-analysis. Since there were none, I chose to follow a qualitative path for my next study, which was a phenomenological study of postpartum depressed women's experiences interacting with their infants during the first year after birth (Beck, 1996a).

In the three qualitative studies that I conducted up to this point in my research program, I repeatedly heard from the depressed mothers how uncaring nurses had been. The next research question centered on exploring the caring experiences of postpartum depressed women with nurses. If some mothers did experience nurses' caring, what was the essence of nurses' caring (Beck, 1995c)? A phenomenological study yielded the answer as I continued along the qualitative path at this next juncture of my research trajectory.

At this time in my research program, I had accumulated rich, insightful data from mothers on postpartum depression, and I was considering conducting an intervention study, thus crossing back over into quantitative methods. To make certain I knew the most current state of the science on postpartum depression before I developed my intervention, I conducted a series of three meta-analyses on the relationship of infant temperament and postpartum depression (Beck, 1996b), predictors of postpartum depression (Beck,1996c), and the effect of postpartum depression on child development (Beck, 1998b). Always trying to get the most from my research studies, I used the findings from the meta-analysis on predictors of postpartum depression to develop the Postpartum Depression Predictors Inventory (Beck, 1998a).

In my earlier qualitative studies, some mothers shared that they had been misdiagnosed with postpartum depression when in fact they were suffering from postpartum-onset panic disorder. At this time, only a few case studies had been published on this postpartum anxiety disorder. My next study led me down a qualitative path to a phenomenological study on panic disorder following childbirth to help tease out subtle differences between this anxiety disorder and postpartum depression (Beck, 1998c). What I have repeatedly discovered in my research trajectory is that qualitative research helps to bring visibility to previously invisible phenomena.

Armed with all the studies included in the meta-analyses I had conducted previously, what became apparent to me were the measurement issues in postpartum depression screening. At that time, only one instrument was available to screen for this mood disorder: the Edinburgh Postnatal

Depression Scale (EPDS; Cox, Holden, & Sagovsky, 1987). In assessing the content validity of the EPDS, I used the results from my series of qualitative studies, and what became clear was that there were major aspects of postpartum depression that were not being measured by the EPDS: loss of self, loneliness, obsessive thinking, loss of control, and mental confusion. Now knowing this limited state of the knowledge on postpartum depression screening, I decided it was premature to conduct an intervention study. What first needed to be done was to develop and test psychometrically a screening scale for postpartum depression, the items of which were derived from the words of the women that I had repeatedly heard in my qualitative studies.

My major roadblock in traveling down this quantitative path was the absence of an instrument development course in my doctoral program. I had no background in instrument development, and so I knew my limitations. In order to develop the Postpartum Depression Screening Scale (PDSS; Beck & Gable, 2002), I consulted with an expert psychometrician, Dr. Robert Gable, at the University of Connecticut. For more than 15 years now, we have collaborated on a number of psychometric studies to determine the reliability, validity, sensitivity, and specificity of the PDSS and its Spanish version (Beck & Gable, 2003). While I was involved in developing and testing the psychometrics of the PDSS, I also conducted a metasynthesis of qualitative studies on postpartum depression (Beck, 2002d). I have often, in my program of research, conducted more than one study at a time. So at this point in my research trajectory, I was going down both a quantitative and a qualitative path.

Sometimes at a junction in a research trajectory, the researcher, fortunately, is at the right place at the right time. That is what happened to me next in 2000. I have already described this in Chapter 2 where I have recounted having been invited to give a keynote address on perinatal anxiety disorders at the Marcé International Society's conference in Christchurch, New Zealand. There I had a fortuitous meeting with Sue Watson, a mother who had started a charitable trust in New Zealand (Trauma and Birth Stress [TABS]) to support women who had experienced birth trauma. For almost 15 years now, with the help of Sue Watson, I have been researching birth trauma and its aftermath. I have conducted six qualitative studies on this topic over the Internet. I followed the qualitative path for a number of years, as you will see. A recruitment notice regarding my research is placed on the TABS website (www.tabs.org.nz). The first of these qualitative studies examined what it was about a birth that could be perceived by mothers as a traumatic childbirth (Beck, 2004a). Next, I conducted another phenomenological study, this time on the resulting posttraumatic stress disorder (PTSD) due to childbirth (Beck, 2004b). In that study, some women briefly mentioned how difficult their child's birthday was to celebrate since it was also a painful reminder of their traumatic childbirth. The anniversary of the birth trauma was the focus of this next study in my sequential research program (Beck, 2006b). After that study, I conducted another phenomenological study to follow up on another topic mothers had mentioned briefly in the early birth trauma studies. This time it was the impact of birth trauma on breastfeeding. It turned out to be a tale of two pathways (Beck & Watson, 2008). For some mothers, their birth trauma facilitated their breastfeeding attempts. These women felt that they had to atone to their infants for the traumatic way they had come into the world, and breastfeeding was the one way they could do that. For other women, their traumatic childbirth took them down a difficult path that hindered their breastfeeding attempts. These women felt violated by their birth trauma and did not want to take the chance their body could be violated again through breastfeeding.

Again, the women in my previous qualitative studies on traumatic birth gave me the idea for another research question to examine: What is the experience of mothers who go on to have a subsequent childbirth after a previous traumatic birth? (Beck & Watson, 2010). Surveying to the results from all my qualitative studies on traumatic childbirth, I recently conducted a metasynthesis on those findings (Beck, 2011).

In the study on the impact of birth trauma on breastfeeding, one woman shared an extremely powerful story of the effect her childhood sexual abuse had had on her labor, delivery, and breastfeeding experiences. I asked her if I could write her story as a case study to help educate clinicians on the distressing repercussions of childhood sexual abuse on a woman's childbearing experience (Beck, 2009a). She responded with an emphatic yes. This mother was thrilled that, hopefully, the traumatic experiences she had suffered through may help prevent another woman from ever experiencing what she had.

During the decade I was traveling down the qualitative path researching various aspects of traumatic childbirth and its resulting PTSD, researchers from various countries around the world had published qualitative studies on postpartum depression in mothers from different cultures. At this juncture in my program of research, I decided it was an appropriate time to modify my original grounded theory study of teetering on the edge using the findings from these published studies (Beck, 2007). The sample of women who had participated in my original grounded theory study (Beck, 1993) was comprised of all Caucasian mothers from the United States. With this modification and a second modification (Beck, 2012), I have extended my grounded theory to include women from other ethnic groups.

While I was conducting my series of qualitative studies on traumatic childbirth and its aftermath, I also finally conducted the intervention study that I had originally envisioned occurring much earlier in my program of research. It was a double blind randomized control trial that investigated the effect on postpartum depressive symptoms of a diet enriched with DHA (omega 3 fatty acids) during pregnancy (Judge, Beck, Durham, McKelvey, & Lammi-Keefe, 2014).

Up to this point in my research trajectory I had not traveled down a mixed methods path, but at this time I believed it was the right choice to make. Here I conducted a mixed methods study examining secondary traumatic stress in labor and delivery nurses (Beck & Gable, 2012). Obstetrical nurses kept saying to me that they were also traumatized by women's traumatic births for which they had been present. My research trajectory was discovering the ever-widening ripple effect of traumatic childbirth. In my next study using a phenomenological approach, I found that fathers, too, were traumatized by being present at their partners' traumatic births (Beck, Driscoll, & Watson, 2013). Yes, the ripple effect was widening even further.

A number of mothers who had participated in my traumatic childbirth studies experienced the frightening obstetrical complication of shoulder dystocia births. Labor and delivery nurses often described shoulder dystocia births as the traumatic births related to their secondary traumatic stress. Trying to get the most out of my qualitative data, next I did a qualitative secondary data analysis comparing the experiences of a shoulder dystocia birth from the perspectives of the nurses and the mothers (Beck, 2013).

Next, as I continued down the qualitative path, it was mothers' experiences of eye movement desensitization reprocessing (EMDR) treatment for their elevated posttraumatic stress symptoms that I focused on (Beck, Driscoll, & Watson, 2013). Women were e-mailing me asking what this treatment was like, so I decided to ask the mothers themselves who had undergone this treatment. Once I completed that study, back to the mixed methods path I went. Prevalence rates were so high with secondary traumatic stress in labor and delivery nurses that I made the decision to now examine this phenomenon in certified nurse-midwives (Beck, LoGiudice, & Gable, 2015).

Currently, I am conducting a phenomenological study on posttraumatic growth in women after a traumatic childbirth. Research is confirming that survivors of traumatic events, such as cancer, experience posttraumatic growth. No research has been done, however, with women who have suffered birth trauma. Hopefully, the results of this study will provide some hope to women suffering with PTSD following childbirth that some positives in their lives can come out of this trauma.

BENEFITS OF META-ANALYSES AND METASYNTHESES IN PLANNING SEQUENTIAL STUDIES

In planning out sequential studies in your research trajectory, a meta-analysis or metasynthesis can be quite helpful in pointing you in the direction of your next study. The reference lists at the end of a meta-analysis and a metasynthesis can be extremely valuable to researchers in identifying relevant published studies in their research areas. Current gaps in the knowledge base in your research area can be identified by the results of these reviews.

Meta-Analysis

Glass (1976) introduced meta-analysis and defined it as "the statistical analysis of a large collection of analysis results from individual studies for the purpose of integrating the findings. It connotes a rigorous alternative to the casual, narrative discussions of research studies which typify our attempts to make sense of the rapidly expanding research literature" (p. 3). Meta-analysis can correct the following weaknesses of traditional literature reviews: (a) the rules used to include studies in the review are rarely stated, (b) there are no systematic methods for resolving contradictory results of the studies in the review, (c) researchers often use their own rules for summarizing the studies, and (d) the researchers' bias can creep into the literature review (Curlette & Cannella, 1985).

Meta-analysis can be quite helpful to researchers in determining the next direction their program of research should take. For instance, if a researcher wants to design an intervention to test, the results of a meta-analysis can assist in narrowing down a significant research problem to be investigated. Take for example my research trajectory. At one point, I was considering developing an intervention for women suffering from postpartum depression, though not knowing what aspect of postpartum depression I should target. I conducted a series of meta-analyses to help in my decision making. One of the meta-analyses was on the effects of postpartum depression on mother–infant interaction during the first year after birth (Beck, 1995b). This meta-analysis certainly can provide a researcher with the rationale for testing an intervention to improve depressed mother–infant interaction over the first year of the infant's life.

Another use of a meta-analysis in a program of research can entail developing an instrument based on the findings. In my program of research, I had conducted two meta-analyses on risk factors for postpartum depression (Beck, 1996c, 2001). The first one was published in 1996. Five years later, I conducted another meta-analysis to update the findings of the 1996 meta-analysis. My next step in my program of research involved a path where I would build on the results of these two meta-analyses. First, based on the 1996 meta-analysis results, I developed the Postpartum Depression Predictors Inventory (PDPI), which was a checklist of eight predictors found to be significantly related to elevated postpartum depressive symptoms (Beck, 1998a). This checklist was designed to be used as an inventory to be completed together by a woman and her health care provider. It was meant to be a starting point for dialogue. After I updated my original meta-analysis in 2001, I discovered that research done in the decade of the 1990s identified an additional five significant risk factors for this devastating mood disorder. Based on these updated findings, I next revised the PDPI to include these five new risk factors (PDPI-Revised; Beck, 2002c). The strength of the development of the PDPI-Revised comes from my two separate meta-analyses. In 2006, I revised the PDPI-Revised from a checklist to a more formal instrument with coding, scoring options, a cutoff score, and its sensitivity and specificity (Table 3.3; Beck, Records, & Rice, 2006; Records, Rice, & Beck, 2007).

• TABLE 3.3 Scoring Directions for the PDPI-Revised

Prenatal Version	Assigning Scores	Total Possible Score per Item	Total Possible Score per Predictor Group	Cumulative Total
Marital status	Range = 0–1		1	1
Single, married, separated, divorced, widowed, partnered	Married/ partnered = 0 All single status = 1	1		
Socioeconomic status	Range = 0–1		1	2
Low, middle, high	Middle or high = 0 Low = 1	1		
Self-esteem	Range = 0–3		3	5
Do you feel good about yourself	Yes = 0 No = 1	1		
Do you feel worthwhile	Yes = 0 No = 1	1		
Do you have good qualities	Yes = 0 No = 1	1		
Prenatal depression	Range = 0–1		1	6
Have you felt depressed during your pregnancy	No = 0 Yes = 1	1		

(continued)

• TABLE 3.3 Scoring Directions for the PDPI-Revised (*continued*)

Prenatal Version	Assigning Scores	Total Possible Score per Item	Total Possible Score per Predictor Group	Cumula-tive Total
If yes, when and how long	Not used			
If yes, how mild or severe	Not used			
Prenatal anxiety	Range = 0–1		1	7
Have you been feeling anxious during your pregnancy	No = 0 Yes = 1	1		
If yes, how long	Not used			
Unplanned/unwanted pregnancy	Range = 0–2		2	9
Was the pregnancy planned	Yes = 0 No = 1	1		
Was the pregnancy unwanted	No = 0 Yes =1	1		
History of previous depression	Range = 0–1		1	10
Before this pregnancy, have you ever been depressed	No = 0 Yes = 1	1		
If yes, when did you ex-perience this depression	Not used			
If yes, have you been under the care of an MD	Not used			
If yes, did the MD prescribe medication	Not used			
Social support partner	Range = 0–4 for each area of part-ner, family, and friends		4	22

(continued)

• TABLE 3.3 Scoring Directions for the PDPI-Revised (*continued*)

Prenatal Version	Assigning Scores	Total Possible Score per Item	Total Possible Score per Predictor Group	Cumula-tive Total
Do you feel you receive adequate emotional support from your partner	Yes = 0 No = 1	1		
Do you feel you can confide in your partner	Yes = 0 No = 1	1		
	Above 2 items = affective partner support			
Do you feel you can rely on your partner	Yes = 0 No = 1	1		
Do you feel you receive adequate instrumental support from your partner	Yes = 0 No = 1	1		
	Above 2 items = partner instrumental support		4	
Family Do you feel you receive adequate emotional support from your family	Yes = 0 No = 1	1		
Do you feel you can confide in your family	Yes = 0 No = 1	1		
	Above 2 items = family effective support			
Do you feel you can rely on your family	Yes = 0 No = 1	1		
Do you feel you receive adequate instrumental support from your family	Yes = 0 No = 1	1		

(*continued*)

• **TABLE 3.3 Scoring Directions for the PDPI-Revised (*continued*)**

Prenatal Version	Assigning Scores	Total Possible Score per Item	Total Possible Score per Predictor Group	Cumula- tive Total
	Above 2 items= family instrumental support		4	
Friends Do you feel you re- ceive adequate emo- tional support from your friends	Yes = 0 No = 1	1		
Do you feel you can confide in your friends	Yes = 0 No = 1	1		
	Above 2 items = friend affective support			
Do you feel you can rely on your friends	Yes = 0 No = 1	1		
Do you feel you re- ceive adequate instru- mental support from your friends	Yes = 0 No = 1	1		
	Above 2 items = friend instrumental support			
Marital/partner satisfaction	Range = 0–3		3	25
Are you satisfied with your marriage or living arrangement	Yes = 0 No = 1	1		
Are you currently ex- periencing any marital/ relationship problems	No = 0 Yes = 1	1		
Are things going well between you and your partner	Yes = 0 No = 1	1		

(continued)

• TABLE 3.3 Scoring Directions for the PDPI-Revised (*continued*)

Prenatal Version	Assigning Scores	Total Possible Score per Item	Total Possible Score per Predictor Group	Cumula- tive Total
Life stress	Range = 0–7		7	**32**
Are you currently experiencing any stressful events in your life such as:				
Financial problems	No = 0 Yes = 1	1		
Marital problems	No = 0 Yes = 1	1		
Death in family	No = 0 Yes = 1	1		
Unemployment	No = 0 Yes = 1	1		
Serious illness in family	No = 0 Yes = 1	1		
Moving	No = 0 Yes = 1	1		
Job change	No = 0 Yes = 1	1		
Postpartum Version				
Child care stress	Range = 0–3		3	**35**
Is the infant experienc- ing any health problems	No = 0 Yes = 1	1		
Are you having prob- lems feeding the baby	No = 0 Yes = 1	1		
Are you having prob- lems with the baby sleeping	No = 0 Yes = 1	1		
Infant temperament	Range = 0–3	3	3	**38**

(continued)

• TABLE 3.3 Scoring Directions for the PDPI-Revised (*continued*)

Prenatal Version	Assigning Scores	Total Possible Score per Item	Total Possible Score per Predictor Group	Cumulative Total
Would you consider the baby irritable	No = 0 Yes = 1	1		
Does the baby cry a lot	No = 0 Yes = 1	1		
Is your baby difficult to console or soothe	No = 0 Yes = 1	1		
Maternity blues	Range 0–1		1	39
Did you experience a period of tearfulness the first week after delivery	No = 0 Yes = 1	1		

PPDI, Postpartum Depression Predictors Inventory.
Reprinted with permission from Beck et al. (2006, pp. 740–742).

Metasynthesis

A metasynthesis is "an interpretive integration of qualitative findings that are themselves interpretive syntheses of data, including the phenomenologies, ethnographies, grounded theories, and other coherent descriptions or explanations of phenomena, events, or cases that are the hallmark findings of qualitative research" (Sandelowski & Barroso, 2007, p. 18). Metasynthesis is a goldmine for evidence-based practice (Beck, 2009c). It can help qualitative research to take its rightful place in the hierarchy of evidence. Thorne et al. (2004) stressed that researchers are obligated to "produce knowledge that is accessible to researchers, clinicians, and the general public that can be translated for practice" (p. 1360). In 1971, Glaser and Strauss warned that results from individual qualitative studies will remain as "respected little islands of knowledge separated from others" (p. 181) unless an approach to building a cumulative body of knowledge is developed.

The aim of conducting a metasynthesis is not to identify similarities of qualitative research studies on a particular topic, but instead, for the researchers to dig deep under the surface of these studies to "emerge with the kernel of a new truth" so that our understanding is enhanced (Paterson,

Thorne, Canam, & Jillings, 2001, p. 111). Metasynthesizers are cautioned to "carefully peel away the surface layers of studies to find their hearts and souls in a way that does the least damage to them" (Sandelowski, Docherty, & Emden, 1997, p. 370).

The most frequently used type of metasynthesis is the integration of findings from a number of qualitative studies on the same topic that have been conducted by different researchers. Another type of metasynthesis involves synthesizing findings from qualitative studies on the same topic, but in this type all the studies have been conducted by the same researcher in his or her program of research (Sandelowski et al., 1997).

Paterson (2013) identified over 20 varying methods of metasynthesis that have been developed over the past two decades. Noblit and Hare's (1988) seminal work on metaethnography is the metasynthesis approach used most frequently to date. Metaethnography is an interpretive metasynthesis method in which primary qualitative research findings are translated into each other. Noblit and Hare's method consists of six overlapping and repeating steps:

1. Deciding on which phenomenon will be studied.
2. Making a choice regarding which qualitative studies will be included in the metasynthesis.
3. Deciding how the studies are related to each other: reciprocal, refutational, or line of argument.
4. Translating the qualitative studies into one another. Noblit and Hare (1988) describe this as "Translations are especially unique syntheses, because they protect the particular, respect holism, and enable comparison. An adequate translation maintains the central metaphors and/or concepts of each account in their relation to other key metaphors or concepts in that account" (p. 28).
5. Synthesizing the translations where the researcher creates a whole that is more than the individual parts imply.
6. Expressing the results in various ways such as written word, plays, art, videos, or music.

Two examples of metaethnographies from my research program on postpartum mood and anxiety disorders are now used to illustrate (a) a metaethnography integrating qualitative studies on postpartum depression conducted by different researchers, and (b) a metaethnography of qualitative studies on traumatic childbirth all conducted by the same researcher, namely, myself. I used Noblit and Hare's method in both of these metasyntheses.

In my postpartum depression metaethnography (Beck, 2002d), I synthesized 18 qualitative studies published between 1990 and 1999. These primary studies were conducted by researchers from the following disciplines: nursing, social work, sociology, psychology, and occupational therapy. These studies took place in various countries: United States, United Kingdom, Australia, and Canada. In translating the findings of one study into the other, four overarching themes emerged that reflected four perspectives involved in women's experiences of postpartum depression: (a) incongruity between expectations and the reality of motherhood, (b) spiraling downward, (c) pervasive loss, and (d) making gains (Figure 3.1).

In my metaethnography of traumatic childbirth and its aftermath (Beck, 2011), I synthesized the results of my six qualitative studies on birth trauma and its resulting PTSD. Two of these studies examined birth trauma itself. One was a phenomenological study (Beck 2004a), and the other was a narrative analysis (Beck, 2006a). The resulting PTSD after traumatic childbirth was the topic of another phenomenological study (Beck, 2004b). The anniversary of birth trauma was the fourth study that also was a phenomenological study (Beck, 2006b). The impact of a traumatic birth on breastfeeding experiences (Beck & Watson, 2008), and subsequent childbirth following a previous

• **FIGURE 3.1 Four Perspectives Involved With Postpartum Depression**

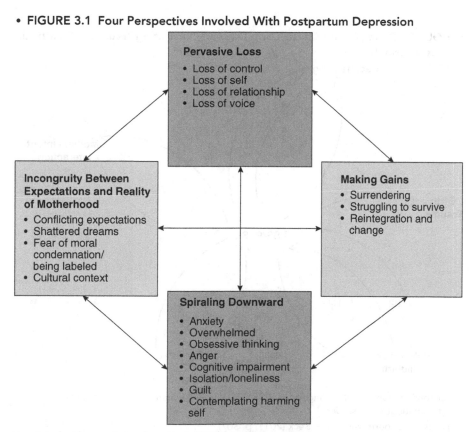

Reprinted with permission from Beck (2002d, p. 461).

birth trauma (Beck & Watson, 2010), were the remaining studies synthesized in this metaethnography. This type of metasynthesis enabled me to see that the aftermath of traumatic childbirth involved a domino effect on multiple aspects of motherhood that I called amplifying causal looping (Figure 3.2). In amplifying causal looping "as consequences become continually causes and causes continually consequences one sees either worsening or improving progressions or escalating severity" (Glaser, 2005, p. 9). Six amplifying feedback loops were the result of traumatic childbirth. Four of these feedback loops were reinforcing (positive direction), and two were balancing (negative direction). The reinforcing feedback loops zeroed in on the adverse effects of posttraumatic stress following birth trauma on women's breastfeeding experiences, mother–infant interactions, yearly anniversary of the traumatic childbirth, and on subsequent childbirth. The two balancing feedback loops involved the healing effects of breastfeeding and subsequent childbirth on posttraumatic stress.

• **FIGURE 3.2** Amplifying Causal Loop Diagram Illustrating Traumatic Childbirth and Its Aftermath

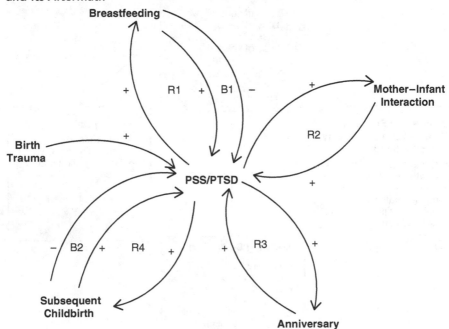

R, reinforcing loops; B, balancing loops; PSS/PTSD, posttraumatic stress symptoms/posttraumatic stress disorder.
Reprinted with permission from Beck (2011, p. 307).

GUIDANCE IN PLANNING SEQUENTIAL STUDIES
WITH SPECIAL POPULATIONS

Nurse researchers have been very generous in sharing with other researchers their experiences, including both challenges and successes, in studying
special populations. These articles can be quite helpful to researchers whose
program of research focuses on one of these special populations. The suggestions of these seasoned researchers can provide valuable guidance in
planning sequential studies in a research trajectory. I have selected some
examples to present in this chapter. The examples highlight research with
end-of-life patients, advanced heart failure patients, ventilator-dependent
patients, acutely ill older patients, older patients in nursing homes, women
in rural settings, and patients in correctional settings.

End of Life

Conducting qualitative interviews with seriously ill patients regarding end
of life can be challenging for researchers. Schulman-Green, McCorkle, and
Bradley (2009–2010) described how they have successfully tailored traditional
interviewing techniques to facilitate the comfort of both the researcher and
the participant in discussing death and dying issues. Due to the challenges
of the debilitated state of the patients, the highly sensitive nature of the interview content, and increased emotionalism, Schulman-Green and colleagues
reported that researchers often prefer to conduct interviews by proxy with
the patients' caregivers. Data obtained from interviews may not be as reliable and valid as data obtained directly from the patients. Schulman-Green
et al. proposed some techniques for conducting qualitative interviews with
seriously ill persons regarding end-of-life issues. Some of their techniques
include:

- Finding a person to recruit who knows participants meeting your sample
  criteria
- Making sure you take adequate time to obtain informed consent
- Developing trust with the participant
- Starting the interview on safer ground and then moving on to more dif-
  ficult topics
- If needed, redirecting the participant
- Allowing the participant to reflect at the end of the interview

    During the recruitment phase of the study, assistance from persons
whom the potential subjects already know and trust, such as a nurse or social

worker, is helpful. Introduction to the study by someone familiar to the patient and protective family members may aid in recruitment. Schulman-Green et al. (2009–2010) stressed that a researcher cannot overlook the importance of taking adequate time in obtaining informed consent for building trust and rapport. Patients who are seriously ill may prefer not to have to read the informed consent, but instead to rely on the researcher's verbal description of the study. When consenting, the researcher should describe the kinds of questions that will be asked during the interview so the patients know what to expect.

One of the biggest challenges for the researcher is advancing the interview to the point where the most delicate topics, such as the prognosis and the dying process, can be discussed with a level of comfort for both the patient and the researcher. Schulman-Green and colleagues (2009–2010) suggested an initial step of gaining a sense of the patient, for example, determining what the patient understands about his or her condition. One of the most fruitful ways to know the patient is to start with an open question, for example, "Can you tell me briefly what has happened since you were first diagnosed?" (p. 95). It is necessary to go slowly through the interview questions to avoid overwhelming the patient. Flexibility is key in order to respect the patient's needs and willingness to discuss such sensitive topics. In ending the interview, the researcher should use a broad question such as "Is there anything else you want to add to help us understand your experience with completing your advance directive?" (p. 98). Schulman-Green and colleagues warn researchers that conducting interviews with this patient population can be emotionally taxing for the interviewer. Self-care is necessary for the well-being of the researcher and the quality of the data. Self-reflection of the interviewer is critical.

Methodological challenges and solutions regarding conducting end-of-life research on the other end of the spectrum, pediatrics, have been described in the literature (Hinds, Burghen, & Pritchard, 2007). Concern stems from not wanting to burden terminally ill children and their parents. From experience with their research, Hinds and colleagues addressed the following challenges:

> (a) Addressing clinicians' concerns about end-of-life studies causing harm to participants; (b) having eligibility periods that were chosen with the clinical situation in mind but are well defined and appropriate for the study aims; (c) using flexible research methods (such as telephone-based interviews) that do not require a face-to-face meeting; (d) needing a backup method to use when documentation of end-of-life care may be missing, incomplete, or difficult to interpret; and (e) addressing generalizability of findings from studies with typical participation rates of 30.5% to 74% of those eligible. (Hinds et al., 2007, p. 460)

Hinds and her research team (2007) have included an eligibility criterion based on health care providers' agreement that the family will not be unduly burdened by approaching them about their end-of-life study. Hinds reported that health care providers chose the do-not-approach-the-family option because the family: (a) did not fully understand their child's clinical situation, (b) were angry, or (c) were too upset to discuss their child's situation. An additional reason health care providers preferred not to refer to families for the studies was that once an end-of-life choice had been decided on, some families quickly left the hospital and took their terminally ill child home.

Because of the varied clinical status of the terminally ill child and the needs of the family, researchers should permit sufficient time for parents to decide on whether or not they want to participate in the study. Hinds suggests a flexible enrollment period around a well-defined event, such as an end-of-life decision or the child's death.

Balancing methodological rigor with the unusual circumstances of terminally ill children and their parents is required. For example, you can permit telephone consent to be tape recorded instead of a parent returning a signed consent. Lastly, Hinds and her research team (2007) recommend a backup method for documenting end-of-life care that may be missing or incomplete in the medical records of the child.

Advanced Heart Failure

Fitzsimons and Strachan (2012) presented an integrative review of 51 studies, and gleaned the methodological and ethical challenges of conducting research with persons who have advanced heart failure and palliative care needs. These authors suggest that an "uneasy alliance" exists between the practice communities of heart failure and palliative care that contributes to some of the challenges for researchers in identifying and gaining access to these patients. Adding to these challenges is the ethical responsibility of researchers to be vigilant to situations that can occur involving persons who may be both physically and mentally vulnerable and near the end of life. Table 3.4 lists the research challenges and potential strategies to counteract these obstacles that Fitzsimons and Strachan summarized in their integrative review.

Ventilator-Dependent Patients in Intensive Care Units (ICUs)

From her own experiences researching care for ventilator-dependent patients in the ICU, Happ shared the methodological challenges of conducting grounded theory in critical care settings and the strategies she implemented

• TABLE 3.4 Methodological Challenges to Research About Palliative
Care for Persons With Heart Failure

Problem	Research Implications	Potential Solutions
Many different terms used to describe heart failure (HF) progression	Lack of clarity in defining sample	Be precise and consistent with terminology. Offer an operational definition that has clearly identified parameters. Adoption of common terminology within HF and palliative communities of practice.
Patients may be unaware of HF diagnosis	Patients cannot be identified as eligible for research	Take an inductive approach, and assess patients' preferences and comfort in using specific terminology. Ensure all research staff have good communication skills and are trained in dealing with the sensitivities of this situation.
Patients may not have had open discussions with doctor regarding prognosis	Ethically challenging to enroll patients in research on palliative care	Avoid using potentially distressing terms in study documentation. Use qualitative methods that have flexibility to adapt to patients' level of insight. Introduce terminology that includes the term "palliative" into open communication with patients with HF early in course of illness.
Lack of prognostic certainty in HF	Difficult to predict which HF patients are eligible for research on palliative care issues	Adopt standardized inclusion criteria based on needs/symptoms versus certain prognosis. Consider other methodologies such as longitudinal studies that provide data over illness trajectory.
Volatile symptoms mean patients have good days and bad days	Research participation may be onerous for patients having a bad day or a bad spell Researchers can misjudge patients' capacity to participate	Use methodology that takes into account patients' psychological and physical condition. Use process consent approach that allows. Build in time and mechanisms that allow for patients' fragility and symptom volatility (i.e., "patient-centered" recruitment and participation activities that are sensitive to the burden of illness).

(continued)

• TABLE 3.4 Methodological Challenges to Research About Palliative Care for Persons With Heart Failure (*continued*)

Problem	Research Implications	Potential Solutions
High levels of mortality in this HF group	High attrition rates due to mortality	Consider the feasibility and ethical implications of contacting bereaved careers to complete.
Clinical teams may be overly protective of patients with advanced HF	Patient recruitment may be inappropriately blocked and selection bias introduced	Include clinical team from earliest stage of proposal development. Work closely with them to develop shared understanding and mutual respect and trust.
Research Ethics Board may judge patients with advanced HF as too vulnerable	Patients with HF denied autonomous participation in research and therefore opportunity to contribute to the development of evidence-based care	Document the rationale for study and realistic cost–benefit analysis. Ensure methodology is sensitive to participants' needs. Articulate the ethical issues clearly, and develop strategies to address these.
Active user involvement is difficult due to patients' symptoms and sensitive nature of subject matter	Patients do not get opportunity to contribute to design and conduct of research	Include patients and family caregivers/carers in the development, design, and implementation of studies. Patient surrogates such as those with successful transplant or carers to provide useful input.

Reprinted with permission from Fitzsimons and Strachan (2012, p. 250).

to overcome these barriers (Happ & Kagan, 2001). These barriers included: (a) cognitive and communication impairments; (b) informed consent, participant accrual, and attrition; and (c) observation and environment. In critical care units with ventilator-dependent patients, these participants are voiceless. The researchers must then consider the question of which data to collect: nonvocal or behavioral data, family members' interpretations, and/or depend on recall from the ICU patients once they are weaned from the ventilator and are well enough to be interviewed. Happ and Kagan listed possible data sources for grounded theory research in critical care settings:

• Informal interviews
• Formal interviews
• Observation (both participant and nonparticipant)

- Clinical record analysis
- Computerized physiologic data/trending
- Relevant policies, procedures, committee reports
- Diaries
- Patient's written communication
- Field notes

Obtaining informed consent from mechanically ventilated ICU patients is another challenge. In addition to available algorithms to screen these voiceless patients regarding their decisional ability to participate in research, Happ and Kagan (2001) offered some tips to fellow researchers, such as sitting close to eye level of the patient when explaining the research study, and limiting the length of time for discussing the study due to fatigue of patients. Attrition due to patient mortality in critical care is a reality with which researchers must contend.

Another methodological challenge in conducting grounded theory research in critical care settings is the number and frequency of disruptions when trying to observe in the ICU. Owing to the fast pace of interactions, the researcher often needs to choose which interactions to observe and track. Videotaping is one option for an unobtrusive method of observation that can yield efficient, accurate records for data analysis. Other suggestions for untapped grounded theory analysis in ICU settings can include longitudinal case analysis and event analysis (Happ & Kagan, 2001).

When choosing a data collection technique for a qualitative research study, it is beneficial to think out of the box. This is exactly what Happ did for one of the studies in her research program on the care of ventilator-dependent ICU patients. The event analysis technique had traditionally been used by ethnographers to capture cultural events such as festivals and rites of passage in the lives of a cultural group. Happ used event analysis to document and analyze critical events and interactions that occur frequently in complex situations in ICUs (Happ, Swigart, Tate, & Crighton, 2004). Happ's research team used diagrams to help analyze the data. Figure 3.3 illustrates a diagram of the sequence of respiratory therapists' behaviors and interactions focusing on beginning a ventilator weaning trial.

Critically Ill Hospitalized Older Adults

Hancock, Chenoweth, and Chang (2003) described the difficulties they encountered in conducting research with acutely ill hospitalized older patients and their satisfaction with the nursing care they received. The first challenge centered on the issues of normal age-related sensory changes in the elderly that can affect communication. Hearing problems and altered level of

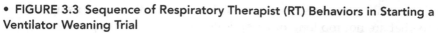

• **FIGURE 3.3** Sequence of Respiratory Therapist (RT) Behaviors in Starting a Ventilator Weaning Trial

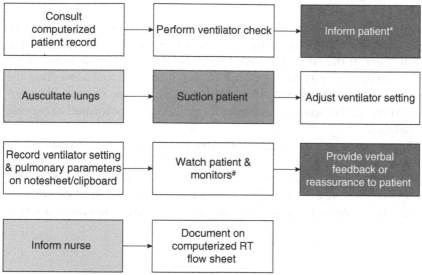

Shaded boxes: These steps were not consistently present. *, If patient is anxious, RT does not inform, but may ask RN to administer anxiolytic medication; #, Surveillance time varies, depending on patient response.

Reprinted with permission from Happ et al. (2004, p. 245).

consciousness can hinder the elderly's receptive ability. Comprehension and rate of information processing can be impaired due to neurological changes. Hancock and colleagues reported that the time needed for acutely ill older patients to complete questionnaires and participate in interviews was longer than that for younger patients.

Another challenge encountered was fatigue. By the time the acutely ill older patient had read and signed the informed consent, completed the demographic information sheet, and been assessed for cognitive functioning, he or she was fatigued before the actual data collection began. Researchers may need to provide time for the subject to rest before being interviewed or completing a questionnaire. Hancock and colleagues (2003) shared that sometimes the patient data collection could not be completed the same day and the researcher needed to come back the next day only to find the patient may have been transferred or become ill or discharged.

If an acutely ill older hospitalized patient is visually impaired, the researchers may need to read the informed consent and questionnaire items or use enlarged print. For some patients with respiratory difficulties, their ability to answer questions is hindered. A cardboard with the Likert response choices on it can be used, and the subjects experiencing respiratory problems can just point to their response. Hancock et al. (2003) suggest using instruments that are not too long or complicated when conducting research with this patient population.

Another reason Hancock and her research team (2003) found why interviews took very long with acutely ill older hospitalized persons was patient loneliness. If the subject received few visitors, the interview was often viewed as an opportunity for social interaction instead of just answering the questionnaire or interview questions. Subjects would often veer off the interview questions and discuss different topics for which they wanted to express their thoughts.

The researchers' ethical responsibility to protect this vulnerable, frail population of older hospitalized adults comes into play throughout the research process. Vigilance not to overburden patients is required. Hancock et al. regularly asked the subjects if they were getting too tired or not feeling well and would rather postpone the rest of the interview until another time.

Older Residents in Nursing Homes

Challenges to conducting research with older persons were also addressed by Hall, Longhurst, and Higginson (2009), but with the older population living in nursing homes. Hall and colleagues' study focused on preserving dignity. Some of the obstacles encountered were finding times to interview the older nursing home residents, staff involvement, maintaining privacy during interviews, and obtaining informed consent. Difficulties with short-term memory loss and cognitive ability hindered the consent process in some participants. Finding time to interview the nursing home residents was often challenging owing to mealtimes, visitors, nursing home activities, hairdresser appointments, and so on.

Hall et al. (2009) were grateful for the help of the nursing home staff with their research, but at times this was problematic. For instance, sometimes the staff emphasized the name of the institution responsible for the research, which would confuse the older residents regarding who would be the researcher. Some thought the researcher was a medical doctor coming to discuss their health.

Monitoring privacy during an interview in a nursing home was yet another challenge. Visitors and staff would come into the resident's room during an interview. Sometimes, the staff had moved an older resident to the dining room or out in the hallway where privacy became a problem. Elderly residents at times preferred to have someone present with them during the interview, which hindered privacy and confidentiality. Hall et al. concluded that the key lessons she and her research team learned were the importance of patience and permitting the older nursing home residents to have as much time as they needed to complete the research process in order to allow the voices of this underrepresented population to be heard in research.

Asian Older Adults

Mehta (2011) described the challenges of conducting research among Asian older adults, specifically when using focus groups. These difficulties included: problems with subjects' access to focus groups sites, need for restrooms to be close by, setting times that fit with eating and naps of the older adults, and gender effect (women not comfortable discussing certain topics with men present). Cognitive impairment with this older population is another potential problem when conducting focus groups. With the elderly, moderators need to be skilled in redirecting the discussion to the topic of the focus group. Asian elders may be hesitant to share their personal experiences in a group setting. Cultural sensitivities, such as respect of the Asian's religion and traditions, are essential to successful focus groups.

Pain Management With Hispanics

McNeill et al. (2003) highlighted issues and strategies that need to be considered when conducting pain management research with Hispanics. In their research, McNeill and colleagues recruited Hispanics to participate in focus groups and one-on-one interviews for the purpose of developing items for a Spanish questionnaire to measure outcomes regarding pain management. Even with a bilingual research assistant, recruitment of potential Hispanic subjects for focus groups was extremely challenging. Unsuccessful attempts occurred to hold focus groups first in a health care facility and then in a Catholic church. Hispanics did not want to discuss private issues, such as pain and illness, in a group. McNeill's research team then tried individual interviews, which were much more successful. One strategy that worked quite well was using telephone interviews with a Spanish-speaking interviewer for recruitment. Individual interviews were found to be a rich source of data with Hispanics.

Rural Populations

Strategies for successful rural research recruitment were addressed by Pribulick, Williams, and Fahs (2010) using their Promoting Heart Health (PHH) in Rural Women study as an illustration. Different challenges were present with recruiting subjects from rural areas as opposed to more densely populated areas. Stepping up efforts and events to recruit subjects may be necessary to overcome barriers in rural areas, such as transportation, isolation, distance, and mistrust of outsiders. Pribulick and colleagues' randomized controlled trial of a community nurse–run intervention to promote heart health was conducted in two rural locations in New York and Virginia. Cardiovascular screening of women was the initial step in this study. To help promote trust of the researchers in these rural communities, no woman was turned away from this screening. Problem solving was required throughout the phase II clinical trial with rural women. Pribulick and her research team needed to broaden their recruitment areas and inclusion criteria in order to facilitate enrollment since there was not such a large pool of potential participants in these rural counties compared to urban areas.

Transportation in rural localities is an obstacle that needs to be overcome. Use of informal networks can be of help but may not always be reliable. If a study is funded, providing transportation for subjects or reimbursing them for their travel expenses can be a solution. Pribulick et al. (2010) also suggest placing data collection sites in the rural localities instead of requiring participants to travel to an urban center. This strategy, however, can result in increased costs and efforts of the research team. In Pribulick and colleagues' clinical trial record-setting flooding rains occurred that destroyed bridges, washed out roads, and damaged homes and businesses, delaying recruitment efforts for several months.

Rural communities may also lag behind urban communities in Internet connections, resulting in challenges in public awareness of recruitment notices for research studies. In their heart health intervention for rural women, Pribulick and her research team used multiple sources to advertise their studies, such as radio interviews, public service announcements, and recruitment notices in newspaper and church bulletins. Utilizing key community liaisons can be critical for successful recruitment in rural communities. The PHH team, for example, developed a close relationship with a church in Virginia that held a health fair every year for that rural community. The research team provided free cardiovascular health screenings at the fair. The health fair organizer and the church health outreach coordinator served as community liaisons for Pribulick and colleagues' study. This research team was successful in the recruitment and retention of their sample of rural women, but the researchers stressed that each barrier to recruitment and retention in rural areas needs to be addressed with careful planning to achieve an adequate sample size and decrease attrition.

Correctional Settings

This chapter ends with a discussion of the unique challenges and solutions for conducting research in correctional settings. Innes (2003) identified the following strategies for conducting research in prisons: (a) garner stakeholders, (b) make sure you have an experienced research collaborator in corrections, (c) obtain technical support from an academic setting, (d) identify possible opportunities and interests that would be of benefit to the mission of the corrections facility, (e) develop a relationship with the institution's internal review board (IRB), and (f) conduct a small pilot study that would be of interest and value to the corrections facility.

Wakai, Shelton, Trestman, and Kesten (2009) illustrated Innes' (2003) strategies with their research on assessing the use of the Corrections Modified Global Assessment of Functioning in evaluating inmates. Wakai and colleagues began by gathering persons who had a stake in the inmates at the correctional facility at which they wanted to conduct their research. These stakeholders had the ability to facilitate change and make a commitment to the research. Examples of some of these stakeholders included the wardens and the director of offender programs and victim services. The stakeholder group met quarterly to give feedback to the researchers on the study activities and to assist in recruiting personnel for focus groups that were one of the main data collection methods.

In the beginning stages of writing the grant for their research, Wakai et al. (2009) met with representatives of the Connecticut Department of Corrections and the University of Connecticut Health Center/Correctional Health Managed Care to identify what the health care needs of the inmates were. Meetings that the research team held with the corrections' IRB helped refine their research protocol. Discussions centered on confidentiality during focus groups, design of the study, and data collection methods.

Apa et al. (2012) also discussed challenges they encountered while conducting research in maximum security prisons and the strategies they found helpful. Table 3.5 outlines the essential components and steps, identified by them, to be taken when conducting research with a department of corrections. Correctional research is developing into a specialty that can help improve the health care of inmates. The obstacles that researchers may encounter are there to ensure the ethical treatment of the inmates.

• TABLE 3.5 Essential Components and Approaches for Conducting Research With a Department of Corrections

Essential Component	Steps to Be Taken	Suggested Approaches
Develop a collaborative research relationship	Know the system.	Review Department of Corrections rules and regulations. Establish early contact with decision makers at the state and prison levels.
	Obtain appropriate permissions.	Obtain approval from Institutional Review Board and from Department of Corrections.
		Obtain OHRP Certification Letter.
	Emphasize mutual goals.	Identify a senior corrections administrator as collaborator/coinvestigator.
		Discuss research interests and aims with faculty superintendents for feedback and modification.
		Clarify benefits to each facility.
Establish the prison contacts	Work with administrative personnel, health care staff, security personnel, and inmates.	Identify key personnel.
		Establish and maintain a professional relationship.
		Emphasize their importance in carrying out the study.
		Keep them fully informed throughout the study.
Maintain rigorous research methods	Accommodate to variations in prison cultures.	Learn how each facility is set up. Know and follow the rules.
		Identify strategies to cope with differences between facilities.
		Manage time to accommodate different recruitment and interview requirements.
	Data collection, maintain inmate's privacy.	Maintain security and confidentiality during interviews and data collection.
		Obtain Certificate of Confidentiality.

Reprinted with permission from Apa et al. (2012, p. 468).

REFERENCES

Apa, Z. L., Bai, R. Y., Mukherejee, D. V., Herzig, C. T., Koenigsmann, C., Low, F. D., & Larson, E. L. (2012). Challenges and strategies for research in prisons. *Public Health Nursing, 29*(5), 467–472.

Beck, A. T., Ward, C. H., Mendelson, M., Mock, J., & Erbaugh, J. (1961). An inventory for measuring depression. *Archives of General Psychiatry, 4*, 561–569.

Beck, C. T. (1992). The lived experience of postpartum depression: A phenomenological study. *Nursing Research, 41*, 166–170.

Beck, C. T. (1993). Qualitative research: The evaluation of its credibility, fittingness and auditability. *Western Journal of Nursing Research, 15*, 263–266.

Beck, C. T. (1995a). Screening methods for postpartum depression. *Journal of Obstetric, Gynecologic, and Neonatal Nursing, 24*, 308–312.

Beck, C. T. (1995b). The effect of postpartum depression of maternal-infant interaction: A meta-analysis. *Nursing Research, 44*, 298–304.

Beck, C. T. (1995c). Perceptions of nurses' caring by mothers experiencing postpartum depression. *Journal of Obstetric, Gynecologic, and Neonatal Nursing, 24*, 819–825.

Beck, C. T. (1996a). Postpartum depressed mothers' experiences interacting with their children. *Nursing Research, 45*(2), 98–104.

Beck, C. T. (1996b). The relationship between postpartum depression and infant temperament: A meta-analysis. *Nursing Research, 45*, 225–230.

Beck, C. T. (1996c). Predictors of postpartum depression: A meta-analysis. *Nursing Research, 45*, 297–303.

Beck, C. T. (1998a). A checklist to identify women at risk for developing postpartum depression. *Journal of Obstetric, Gynecologic, and Neonatal Nursing, 27*, 39–46.

Beck, C. T. (1998b). Effects of postpartum depression on child development: A meta-analysis. *Archives of Psychiatric Nursing, 12*, 12–20.

Beck, C. T. (1998c). Postpartum onset of panic disorder. *Image: Journal of Nursing Scholarship, 30*, 131–135.

Beck, C. T. (2001). Predictors of postpartum depression: An update. *Nursing Research, 50*, 275–285.

Beck, C. T. (2002a). Releasing the pause button: Mothering twins during the first year of life. *Qualitative Health Research, 12*, 593–608.

Beck, C. T. (2002b). Mothering multiples: A meta-synthesis of the qualitative research. *MCN: The American Journal of Maternal Child Nursing, 27*, 214–221.

Beck, C. T. (2002c). Revision of the Postpartum Depression Predictors Inventory. *Journal of Obstetric, Gynecologic, and Neonatal Nursing, 31*, 394–402.

Beck, C. T. (2002d). Postpartum depression: A meta-synthesis of qualitative research. *Qualitative Health Research, 12*, 453–472.

Beck, C. T. (2004a). Birth trauma: In the eye of the beholder. *Nursing Research, 53*, 28–35.

Beck, C. T. (2004b). Post-traumatic stress disorder due to childbirth: The aftermath. *Nursing Research, 53*, 216–224.

Beck, C. T. (2006a). Pentadic cartography: Mapping birth trauma narratives. *Qualitative Health Research, 16*, 453–466.

Beck, C. T. (2006b). The anniversary of birth trauma: Failure to rescue. *Nursing Research, 55*, 381–390.

Beck, C. T. (2007). Exemplar: Teetering on the edge: A continually emerging theory of postpartum depression. In P. L. Munhall (Ed.) *Nursing research: A qualitative perspective* (4th ed., pp. 273–292). Sudbury, MA: Jones & Bartlett.

Beck, C. T. (2009a). An adult survivor of childhood sexual abuse and her breastfeeding experience: A case study. *MCN: American Journal of Maternal Child Nursing, 34,* 91–97.

Beck, C. T. (2009b). The arm: There's no escaping the reality for mothers caring for their children with obstetric brachial plexus injuries. *Nursing Research, 58,* 237–245.

Beck, C. T. (2009c). Metasynthesis: A goldmine for perioperative evidence-based practice. *AORN Journal, 90,* 701–710.

Beck, C. T. (2011). A metaethnography of traumatic childbirth and its aftermath: Amplifying causal looping. *Qualitative Health Research, 21,* 301–311.

Beck, C. T. (2012). Exemplar: Teetering on the edge: A second grounded theory modification. In P. L. Munhall (Ed.), *Nursing research: A qualitative perspective* (5th ed., pp. 257–284). Sudbury, MA: Jones & Bartlett Publishers.

Beck, C. T. (2013). The obstetric nightmare of shoulder dystocia: A tale from two perspectives. *MCN: The American Journal of Maternal Child Nursing, 38,* 34–40.

Beck, C. T., & Gable, R. K. (2000). Postpartum Depression Screening Scale: Development and psychometric testing. *Nursing Research, 49,* 272–282.

Beck, C. T., & Gable, R. K. (2001a). Further validation of the Postpartum Depression Screening Scale. *Nursing Research, 50,* 155–164.

Beck, C. T., & Gable, R. K. (2001b). Comparative analysis of the performance of the Postpartum Depression Screening Scale with two other depression instruments. *Nursing Research, 50,* 242–250.

Beck, C. T., & Gable, R. K. (2002). *Postpartum Depression Screening Scale Manual.* Los Angeles, CA: Western Psychological Services.

Beck, C. T., & Gable, R. K. (2003). Postpartum Depression Screening Scale—Spanish Version. *Nursing Research, 52,* 296–306.

Beck, C. T., & Gable, R. K. (2005). Screening performance of the Postpartum Depression Screening Scale Spanish Version. *Journal of Transcultural Nursing, 16,* 331–338.

Beck, C. T., & Gable, R. K. (2012). A mixed methods study of secondary traumatic stress in labor and delivery nurses. *Journal of Obstetric, Gynecologic, and Neonatal Nursing, 41,* 747–760.

Beck, C. T., Driscoll, J. W., & Watson, S. (2013). *Traumatic childbirth.* New York, NY: Routledge.

Beck, C. T., Gable, R. K., Sakala, C., & Declercq, E. R. (2011a). Posttraumatic stress disorder in new mothers: Results from a two-stage U.S. national survey. *Birth, 38,* 216–227.

Beck, C. T., Gable, R. K., Sakala, C., & Declercq, E. R. (2011b). Postpartum depression in new mothers: Results from a two-stage U.S. national survey. *Journal of Midwifery and Women's Health, 56,* 427–435.

Beck, C. T., Kurz, B., & Gable, R. K. (2012a). Concordance and discordance of the Postpartum Depression Screening Scale (PDSS) and the Patient Health Questionnaire-9 (PHQ-9) in an ethnically diverse sample. *Journal of Social Service Research, 38,* 439–450.

Beck, C. T., LoGiudice, J., & Gable, R. K. (2015). Shaken belief in the birth process: A mixed methods study of secondary traumatic stress in certified nurse-midwives. *Journal of Midwifery & Women's Health, 60,* 16–23.

Beck, C. T., Records, K., & Rice, M. (2006). Further validation of the Postpartum Depression Predictors Inventory-Revised. *Journal of Obstetric, Gynecologic, and Neonatal Nursing, 35,* 735–745.

Beck, C. T., Reynolds, M., & Rutowski, P. (1992). Maternity blues and postpartum depression. *Journal of Obstetric, Gynecologic, and Neonatal Nursing, 21,* 287–293.

Beck, C. T., & Watson, S. (2008). The impact of birth trauma on breastfeeding: A tale of two pathways. *Nursing Research, 57,* 228–236.

Beck, C. T., & Watson, S. (2010). Subsequent childbirth after a previous traumatic birth. *Nursing Research, 59,* 241–249.

Cox, J. L., Holden, J. M., & Sagovsky, R. (1987). Detection of postpartum depression. Development of the 10-item Edinburgh Postnatal Depression Scale. *British Journal of Psychiatry, 150,* 782–786.

Curlette, W., & Cannella, K. (1985). Going beyond the narrative summarization of research findings: The meta-analysis approach. *Research in Nursing & Health, 8,* 293–301.

Fitzsimons, D., & Strachan, P. H. (2012). Overcoming the challenges of conducting research with people who have advanced heart failure and palliative care needs. *European Journal of Cardiovascular Nursing, 11*(2), 248–254.

Glaser, B. G. (2005). *The grounded theory perspective III: Theoretical coding.* Mill Valley, CA: Sociology Press.

Glaser, B. G., & Strauss, A. L. (1971). *Status passage.* Chicago, IL: Aldine-Atherton.

Glass, G. (1976). Primary, secondary, and meta-analysis of research. *The Educational Researcher, 5,* 3–8.

Hall, S., Longhurst, S., & Higginson, I. J. (2009). Challenges to conducting research with older people living in nursing homes. *BMC Geriatrics, 9* (1), 38.

Hancock, K., Chenoweth, L., & Chang, E. (2003). Challenges in conducting research with acutely ill hospitalized older patients. *Nursing and Health Sciences, 5,* 253–259.

Happ, M. B., & Kagan, S. H. (2001). Methodological considerations for grounded theory research in critical care settings. *Nursing Research, 50*(3), 188–192.

Happ, M. B., Swigart, V., Tate, J., & Crighton, M. H. (2004). Event analysis techniques. *Advances in Nursing Science, 27*(3), 239–248.

Hegedus, K., & Beck, C.T. (2012). Development and psychometric testing of the Postpartum Depression Screening Scale: Hungarian version. *International Journal for Human Caring, 16,* 54–58.

Hinds, P. S., Burghen, E. A., & Pritchard, M. (2007). Conducting end-of-life studies in pediatric oncology. *Western Journal of Nursing Research, 29*(4), 448–465.

Innes, C. A. (2003). *Learning lessons and lessons learned: The National Institute of Justice's Research Demonstration Project Strategy.* Paper prepared for the Annual Meetings of the Academy of Criminal Justice Sciences, Boston, MA.

Judge, M. P., Beck, C. T., Durham, H., McKelvey, M. M., & Lammi-Keefe, C. (2014). Pilot trial evaluating maternal DHA consumption during pregnancy decreases postpartum depressive symptomatology. *International Journal of Nursing Sciences, 1*(4), 339–345.

McNeill, J. A., Sherwood, G., Starck, P., Disnard, G., Rodriguez, T., & Palos, G. (2003). Design strategies in pain management research with Hispanics. *Hispanic Health Care International, 2*(2), 73–80.

Mehta, K. K. (2011). The challenges of conducting focus group research among Asian older adults. *Ageing and Society, 31,* 408–421.

Noblit, S. W., & Hare, R. D. (1988). *Meta-ethnography: Synthesizing qualitative studies.* Newbury Park, CA: SAGE.

Paterson, B. (2013). Metasynthesis. In C. T. Beck (Ed.), *Routledge international handbook of qualitative nursing research* (pp. 331–346). New York, NY: Routledge.

Paterson, B. L., Thorne, S. E., Canam, C., & Jillings, C. (2001). *Meta-study of qualitative health research.* Thousand Oaks, CA: SAGE.

Pribulick, M., Williams, I. C., & Fahs, P. S. (2010). Strategies to reduce barriers to recruitment and participation. *Online Journal of Rural Nursing and Health Care, 10*(1), 22–33.

Records, K., Rice, M., & Beck, C. T. (2007). Psychometric assessment of the Postpartum Depression Predictors Inventory-Revised. *Journal of Nursing Measurement, 15,* 189–202.

Sandelowski, M., & Barroso, J. (2007). *Handbook for synthesizing qualitative research.* New York, NY: Springer Publishing Company.

Sandelowski, M., Docherty, S., & Emden, C. (1997). Qualitative meta-synthesis: Issues and techniques. *Research in Nursing & Health, 20*(4), 265–271.

Schulman-Green, D., McCorkle, R., & Bradley, E. H. (2009–2010). Tailoring traditional interviewing techniques for qualitative research with seriously ill patients about the end-of-life: A primer. *Omega, 60*(1), 89–102.

Thorne, S., Jensen, L., Kearney, M. H., Noblit, G., & Sandelowski, M. (2004). Qualitative metasynthesis: Reflections on methodological orientation and ideological agenda. *Qualitative Health Research, 14*(10), 1342–1365.

Wakai, S., Shelton, D., Trestman, R. L., & Kesten, K. (2009). Conducting research in corrections: Challenges and solutions. *Behavioral Sciences and the Law, 27,* 743–752.

Options Available for Developing a Research Program

Do not go where the path may lead, go instead where there
is no path and leave a trail.
—*Ralph Waldo Emerson*

QUALITATIVE RESEARCH CAN BE A GOLD MINE IN DEVELOPING PROGRAMS OF RESEARCH

Van Manen (1990), in his call for action, stated, "Ask not what qualitative research can do for you; ask what qualitative research can do 'with' you and what you can do better with qualitative research" (p. 45). Using findings from qualitative studies that a researcher has previously conducted can be a fruitful and valuable path one can choose to further a program of research. The fact that a qualitative study is completed does not necessarily mean a researcher is done with those data and will not use them again. Putting your qualitative data to use again, but this time in a different study, can jump-start a research program.

Instrument Development

Results from qualitative studies can provide a rich and fruitful source of items for an instrument developer. Indicators derived from qualitative data can result in items that are unique in reflecting a person's experience of the topic being measured by an instrument (Fleury, 1993). Imle and Atwood (1988) caution instrument developers about the challenges they may face in trying to preserve the meaning of qualitative data. Keeping both the language and the expressions that the study participants used in their interviews is key to developing meaningful scale items.

In developing the Postpartum Depression Screening Scale (PDSS; Beck & Gable, 2002), I used data from three qualitative studies I had previously conducted. One study was a grounded theory study (Beck, 1993), and two studies were phenomenological studies (Beck, 1992, 1996). In developing individual items for the PDSS, I started by reviewing all the transcripts of the data from these three studies. To make sure I kept the qualitative meaning of the data, I wrote each scale item to correspond with a specific verbatim quote from the transcripts of the participants' interviews. Table 4.1 illustrates how five items of the PDSS were developed using this process (Beck & Gable, 2001a).

Qualitative studies are also invaluable as a method to assess the content validity of an existing instrument (Tilden, Nelson, & May, 1990). In my research program, I had never envisioned developing an instrument, but it became the path I followed after I had assessed the content validity of the Edinburgh Postnatal Depression Scale (EPDS; Cox, Holden, & Sagovsky, 1987). At that time in my research trajectory I was searching for a screening scale for postpartum depression that I could use in a future quantitative study. There was only one published postpartum depression screening scale I could locate, and that was the EPDS. I assessed its content validity using my series of qualitative studies on postpartum depression. What I found was that there were components of postpartum depression that were not measured by the EPDS. Those missing features were loss of control, loneliness, unrealness, irritability, fear of going crazy, obsessive thinking, difficulty concentrating,

• **TABLE 4.1 Development of Selected Postpartum Depression Screening Scale (PDSS) Items From Qualitative Data**

Quote	Item
"I was so anxious about caring for the baby, even about the littlest of things."	I got anxious over even the littlest things that concerned my baby.
"I didn't know who I had become anymore. It was as if I was a stranger to myself."	I felt as though I had become a stranger to myself.
"Even though I was exhausted, I couldn't fall asleep even when my baby was sleeping."	I had trouble sleeping even when my baby was asleep.
"I had such a hard time even making a simple decision like which outfit I was going to put the baby in."	I had a difficult time making even a simple decision.
"I felt such guilt because I couldn't love my baby like I knew I should."	I felt guilty because I could not feel as much love for my baby as I should.

and loss of self. Knowing that the items on a screening scale should cast a net wide enough to assess the gamut of symptoms a new mother could experience with postpartum depression, I decided to develop the PDSS using the qualitative data from my studies to create the items. A series of two psychometric studies were conducted to develop and test the PDSS.

Once I had made the decision to develop an instrument, I consulted with Robert Gable, EdD, who is an expert in instrument development (Gable & Wolf, 1993; McCoach, Gable, & Madura, 2013). For over 15 years now, we have worked together on the PDSS and studies using this screening scale. In our first psychometric study, the preliminary PDSS was developed and its reliability assessed with a sample of 525 mothers (Beck & Gable, 2000). The preliminary 56 items were reduced to the final 35 items. The items with low reliability levels were deleted. The final version of the PDSS consists of seven dimensions of symptoms with five items per dimension.

The second psychometric study assessed the reliability and validity of the final 35-item version of the PDSS with a sample of 150 new mothers (Beck & Gable, 2001b, 2001c). The reliability coefficient for the data from the total PDSS was $r = 0.96$ with the dimension scale alphas ranging from 0.80 to 0.91. The validity and screening performance of the PDSS were compared with those of two depression instruments: the EPDS and a general depression scale, the Beck Depression Inventory-II (Beck, Steer, & Brown, 1996). As can be seen in Figure 4.1 when assessing incremental validity, the PDSS offered additional power to predict assignment of women to the depressed

• **FIGURE 4.1** Hierarchical Regression of the Diagnosis of Postpartum Depression on the BDI-II, EPDS, and PDSS

Variables	Postpartum Depression Diagnosis	BDI-II	EPDS	PDSS	R	R^2	Increase R^2	Beta
BDI-III	.62				.62	.38	.38**	.15
EPDS	.59	.82			.64	.41	.03*	.01
PDSS	.70	.81	.79		.71	.50	.09**	.56
Means	1.31	10.03	6.75	64.57				
Standard deviation	.46	7.25	4.93	23.62				

* p=.039
** p< .0001

BDI-II, Beck Depression Inventory-II; EPDS, Edinburgh Postnatal Depression Scale; PDSS, Postpartum Depression Screening Scale.

Reprinted with permission from Beck and Gable (2001b, p. 159).

or nondepressed groups, even after the predictive abilities of the EPDS and the BDI-II were statistically removed. The PDSS was the only scale out of the three instruments that identified 17% of the mothers in the sample of 150 women diagnosed with major postpartum depression (Beck & Gable, 2001b). Why was the PDSS able to correctly identify these mothers? The difference had to do with the items related to sleeping disturbances, anxiety, and cognitive impairment. The benefits of items based on my qualitative research studies came out loud and clear. In Table 4.2 are some publications of studies in which the PDSS has been translated into other languages and psychometrically tested.

• **TABLE 4.2 Publications of Studies in Which Postpartum Depression Screening Scale (PDSS) Was Translated Into Other Languages**

Author (Year)	Title	Country
Vittayanont, Liabsuetrakul, and Pitanupong (2006)	Development of Postpartum Depression Scale: A Thai version for screening postpartum depression	Thailand
Cantilino et al. (2007)	Translation, validation and cultural aspects of Postpartum Depression Screening Scale in Brazilian Portuguese	Brazil
Karacam and Kitis (2008)	Postpartum Depression Screening Scale: Its reliability and validity for the Turkish population	Turkey
Clarke (2008)	Validation of two postpartum depression screening scales with a sample of First Nations and Metis women	Canada
Zubaran et al. (2009)	Validation of a screening instrument for postpartum depression in Southern Brazil	Brazil
Zubaran et al. (2010a)	Correlation between postpartum depression and health status	Brazil
Zubaran et al. (2010b)	The Portuguese version of the Postpartum Depression Screening Scale-Short Form	Brazil
Quelopana and Champion (2010)	Validation of the Postpartum Depression Screening Scale-Spanish version in women from Arica, Chile	Chile
Pereira et al. (2010)	Portuguese version of the Postpartum Depression Screening Scale	Portugal

(continued)

• **TABLE 4.2 Publications of Studies in Which Postpartum Depression Screening Scale (PDSS) Was Translated Into Other Languages (*continued*)**

Author (Year)	Title	Country
Zubaran and Foresti (2011)	Investigating quality of life and depressive symptoms in the postpartum period	Brazil
Li, Liu, Zhang, Wang, and Wiaofang (2011)	Chinese version of the Postpartum Depression Screening Scale	China
Maia et al. (2011)	Epidemiology of perinatal depression in Portugal	Portugal
Quelopana, Champion, and Reyes-Rubilar (2011)	Factors associated with postpartum depression in Chilean women	Chile
Quelopana (2012)	Violence against women and postpartum depression: The experience of Chilean women	Chile
Kossakowska (2012)	A Polish adaptation and psychometric evaluation of the Postpartum Depression Screening Scale	Poland
Zubaran and Foresti (2013)	Correlation between breastfeeding self-efficacy and maternal postpartum depression in Southern Brazil	Brazil
Pereira et al. (2013)	Short forms of the Postpartum Depression Screening Scale: As accurate as the original form	Portugal
Lara, Navarrete, Navarro, and Le (2013)	Evaluation of the psychometric measures for the Postpartum Depression Screening Scale—Spanish version for Mexican women	Mexico

Secondary Qualitative Data Analysis

Back in 1979, Sharrock and Anderson were in favor of mining the rich vein of qualitative data studies. Sandelowski (1997a) is also in favor of secondary qualitative data analysis, as illustrated by her quote: "Our notion of programs of research ought also to include efforts to make the most of data already collected, such as the deliberate pursuit of multiple analytic paths within a data set that are later synthesized as well as secondary analysis and meta-synthesis projects combining data sets or findings from different studies" (p. 221).

Secondary analysis of quantitative data is a common, accepted approach for maximizing the use of large national data sets. Secondary analysis of qualitative data sets is now coming into its own and becoming a respected approach. Qualitative researchers know all too well the significant time, energy, and resources that are necessary to conduct a qualitative study. Qualitative researchers began to ask themselves why not conduct a secondary analysis with their typical voluminous data sets just like the quantitative researchers do. The momentum for secondary qualitative data analysis is ever increasing. Thorne (2013) warns that "a coherent body of methodological guidance is just beginning to emerge" (p. 394).

Although the benefits of secondary qualitative data analysis can be considerable, there are some methodological challenges researchers need to contend with: (a) nature of existing data, (b) ethical issues, and (c) matters of voice and representation (Thorne, 2013). In considering the first challenge, the researcher needs to determine the degree to which the data from the original qualitative study are amenable to secondary analysis. How close is the fit between the new research question and the existing qualitative data set? Even if the fit is good, researchers also need to assess the completeness and quality of the original qualitative data set and their access to the data and primary research team (Hinds, Vogel, & Clarke-Steffen, 1997). The second challenge concerns the ethical aspect of the use of the existing qualitative data set. Was informed consent given for reuse of the data? What about confidentiality? The researcher who performs the secondary qualitative data analysis may unwittingly violate confidentiality that the original researcher avoided. The third challenge concerns matters of voice and representation. As Thorne (2013) warns, there are interpretive hazards that may jeopardize the results of the secondary qualitative analysis. Qualitative research involves some degree of interpretation. The original researcher interpreted the primary data. Next, a researcher conducting a secondary analysis adds another layer of interpretation. Errors in interpretation can occur in the primary study and then secondary analysis can compound or exaggerate these misinterpretations.

Thorne proposed the following five approaches to secondary qualitative data analysis:

1. Analytic expansion involves using data from one of the researcher's original studies to answer a new research question or analyze the data at a different level.
2. In retrospective interpretation, the original database is reanalyzed to answer new research questions that had not been thoroughly investigated.
3. Armchair induction focuses on theory development using the original dataset.
4. In amplified sampling, more than one existing database is compared with another database to develop a broader theory.
5. Cross-validation involves using original databases to support or not support new findings.

Sandelowski (1997b) observed that as qualitative nurse researchers "we have become inveterate data collectors, having been imbued with the idea that research means collecting new data" (p. 129). Our mind set is changing. Also Thorne (2013) states "clearly there is a great deal more that we can do with what we already possess" (p. 403).

Secondary qualitative data analysis can be done with more than one data set at a time. An example from my research program illustrates this as an option for researchers in developing their research trajectories. Beck (2013) compared and contrasted the experiences of a shoulder dystocia birth from the perspectives of the mothers and of the labor and delivery nurses (Table 4.3). In the first original study, Beck (2009) conducted a phenomenological study of mothers' experiences of caring for their infants with a brachial plexus injury as a result of a shoulder dystocia birth. The second original study was a mixed methods study of secondary traumatic stress in labor and delivery nurses (Beck & Gable, 2012). The data from the qualitative

• TABLE 4.3 Comparison of the Traumatic Experiences of Shoulder Dystocia: The Obstetric Nightmare

Mothers' Perspectives	Nurses' Perspectives
"The labor felt like I was assaulted for a prolonged time and like my child was assaulted at birth."	"I felt like I was part of a gang rape."
"If only I could have fought back then, but I was in a helpless position myself."	"I felt helpless at the birth because everything we tried didn't work."
"I was screaming 'Please let my baby be okay, please God let my baby be okay.'"	"I was silently praying God, please save this baby."
"I never got congratulated when my baby was born. I wasn't even told there was an injury."	"The baby's head delivered and then there was silence. The nurses in the room gave each other 'the look.'"
"The people who harm your baby for life just walk away with no apology and often no support." (Beck, 2009, p. 241)	"Feelings of regret that we (the nurses) didn't speak up. Scared because we were concerned about this baby's prognosis, if it would come back as a lawsuit."
"I almost feel as if a part of me died on the day I gave birth. Isn't that ironic?" (Beck, 2009, p. 240)	"Immediately I felt numb. I was in shock."

Reprinted with permission from Beck (2013, p. 36).

strand of this mixed methods study, where the nurses described shoulder dystocia deliveries as the traumatic births they had attended, were used in the secondary data analysis. Content analysis (Krippendorff, 2013) was used to compare these two qualitative data sets and investigate the new research question in this qualitative secondary analysis: "What are the similarities and differences in mothers' and labor and delivery nurses' experiences of shoulder dystocia births?" (p. 35).

What led me to turn down this path of secondary qualitative data analysis in my research program? It happened to be two phrases that I heard time and again in my two original qualitative studies. Mothers repeatedly shared that they felt as if they had been raped on the delivery table during their shoulder dystocia births (Beck, 2009). Nurses, on the other hand, often expressed that they felt like they had participated in a gang rape while the labor and delivery team tried to deliver the infant's shoulders (Beck, 2013). This was so striking to me that I decided I needed to further analyze these two datasets in order to unearth a more thorough comparison of the perspectives of these two groups. This secondary qualitative data analysis revealed four themes: (a) in the midst of the obstetric nightmare; (b) reeling from the trauma that just transpired; (c) enduring heartbreak: the heavy toll on mothers; and (d) haunted by memories: the heavy toll on nurses. Table 4.3 provides a glimpse of the outcome of using these two qualitative data sets to answer a new research question.

Examples of secondary qualitative data analysis from two other nurse researchers' programs of research are presented here. Hall (2000) performed a secondary qualitative analysis of 20 narratives of urban low-income childhood abuse survivors who were recovering cocaine misusers. The research questions in the initia qualitative study were:

- What central beliefs do women childhood abuse survivors associate with childhood abuse experiences? In what ways are they associated?
- How do these women relate the context of abuse events, especially dynamics within the family of origin, to these central beliefs and experiences?
- Do women childhood abuse survivors recognize early life events and perceptions as relevant to current life difficulties, especially substance use problems? If so, in what ways are they related? (p. 447)

The focus of Hall's secondary analysis was on learning and work difficulties in women childhood abuse survivors, and it revealed five broad categories: school as problematic, lack of adult life skills, problems with academic and health literacy, legitimate and illicit forms of work, and means of help.

In Morse's program of research on suffering, one of her studies was a qualitative secondary analysis of videotapes of trauma room care (Morse & Pooler, 2002). In building a research trajectory, researchers should not limit themselves to secondary qualitative analysis with just data from interviews, but instead think out of the box as Morse had done. She used data from videotaping. In the original qualitative study, Morse used qualitative ethology to examine videotaped interactions between patients, family members, and nurses in 193 trauma scenarios in three emergency departments. Ethology is a qualitative research design that identifies complex behaviors in the natural setting by means of observation and description. In 88 of the 193 videotaped trauma scenarios, family members were present in the trauma room. Secondary qualitative data analysis focused on verbal and nonverbal interactions among nurses, patients, and their family members in these 88 cases. Morse's model of suffering was the framework used to code data relating to types of triadic care given according to categories of enduring or emotional suffering (Table 4.4).

Happ and her research team recently conducted a secondary analysis of data from her ethnographic study in the intensive care unit (ICU), where she reported that anxiety and agitation occurred often in mechanically ventilated patients (Tate, Dabbs, Hoffman, Milbrandt, & Happ, 2012). Data from 30 critically ill patients, who were weaned from prolonged mechanical ventilation, included observations, interviews, and medical record data. From this secondary analysis, Happ constructed the Anxiety/Agitation in Mechanical Ventilation Model, which depicts the multidimensional aspects of anxiety and agitation recognition and management. The model incorporates both patient and clinician perspectives.

Grounded Theory Modification

In grounded theory, modification never stops (Glaser, 2001). Once a grounded theory study is completed, it should not just lie dormant. As new data are collected by the grounded theorist or as new qualitative studies are published in the literature, these data can be used to modify the original substantive theory. "All is data" for grounded theorists (Glaser, 2001, p. 145). Data from new literature are compared as simply additional data yielding new properties of categories (Glaser, 1998). The grounded theorist can increase the scope of the original substantive theory by making conscious choices of groups for comparison (Glaser & Strauss, 1967). Glaser (1998) cautions that it is not persons who are categorized but the behavior they engage in. Maximizing differences among these compared groups is a powerful approach for extending the substantive theory.

In 1993, I published my original grounded theory study of postpartum depression, "Teetering on the Edge." It was a four-stage process whereby women suffering from postpartum depression grappled with the basic social psychological problem of loss of control. The four stages in

• TABLE 4.4 Types of Triadic Caregiving According to Categories of States of Enduring and Releasing for Patients and Their Families

Nurse–Patient–Family Behaviors and Interactions					
Descriptors	Families Learning to Endure	Patients Failing to Endure	Family Emotionally Suffering and Patient Enduring	Patient and Family Enduring	Resolution of Enduring
Schematic representation					
Patient's state	Unresponsive or sedated	Distressed; afraid; in pain	Scared or anxious	Quiet and in control	Stable and waiting
Direction of care (nurse)	Not patient-led; task oriented	Follows patient's cues; task oriented	Patient-led; works through patients to help family	Patient-led; patient tries to enable family enduring	Tasks minimal; family may leave bedside
Time orientation (patient)	Present	Present	Present	Present	Near future
Nurse's focus	On patient	On patient	On family	On family and patient	On completing care

(continued)

• **TABLE 4.4 Types of Triadic Caregiving According to Categories of States of Enduring and Releasing for Patients and Their Families (continued)**

Nurse–Patient–Family Behaviors and Interactions

Descriptors	Families Learning to Endure	Patients Failing to Endure	Family Emotionally Suffering and Patient Enduring	Patient and Family Enduring	Resolution of Enduring
Family's state	Enter enduring, releasing may break through	Enduring	Emotionally suffering (leave or turn away to hide releasing)	Quiet and in control	Initially release tension; bored or busy making arrangements
Family's focus	On nurse, watching; model/echo nurse's talk	On patient	On self	On patient	On context
Time orientation (family)	Immediate present Lose sense of time	Immediate present	Near future Recognize ramifications	Present	Near future
Interactions (nurse)	Informs about patient's condition; encourages learning to endure	Gives minimal explanation and information	Watches; encourages enduring and monitors interactions	Verbal recognition and promotes enduring	Chats; may discuss feelings of patient or family members

Reprinted with permission from Morse and Pooler (2002, p. 246).

order were: Encountering Terror, Dying of Self, Struggling to Survive, and Regaining Control. All the participants in this study were Caucasian. In 2007, I first modified this substantive theory, increasing its scope to include the behavior of non-Caucasian mothers from other countries than the United States (Beck, 2007). At that time, I located 10 qualitative studies that had been published in which postpartum depression had been examined in women from other cultures. Examples of some of these countries included Australia, India, and China.

Five years after this first modification of Teetering on the Edge, 17 new transcultural qualitative studies on postpartum depression had been published. I incorporated the data from these new studies as additional data for constantly comparing with the first modification (Beck, 2012). Data from these new countries included Sweden, New Zealand, Indonesia, Democratic Republic of Congo, United Arab Emirates, Ethiopia, and Taiwan. With the help of data from these newly published qualitative studies, continuing modifications of Teetering on the Edge were made. For the categories pertaining to each of the four stages of postpartum depression, the countries other than the United States were listed where data supported and endorsed the categories (Figure 4.2). New categories were discovered in this second modification

- **FIGURE 4.2 Second Modification of Teetering on the Edge: Stage 1**

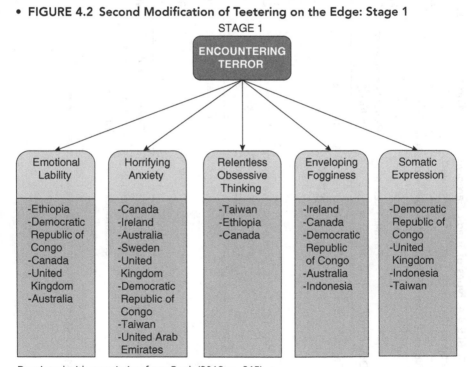

Reprinted with permission from Beck (2012, p. 265).

(Beck, 2012). For example, the first stage of Teetering on the Edge was Encountering Terror. Included in this first stage were four categories: emotional lability, horrifying anxiety, relentless obsessive thinking, and enveloping fogginess. When this substantive theory was enhanced with data from the countries of the Democratic Republic of Congo, Indonesia, Taiwan, and women from Bangladesh living in the U.K., a new category was added to Stage 1: somatic expressions. Mothers in these countries used physical symptoms to describe their postpartum depression. A mother from Indonesia described tiredness in her heart, while a woman from the Democratic Republic of Congo complained of stomach pains and aches in her lower abdomen. A mother from Taiwan explained that she lost strength in her arms and legs, while depressed mothers from India often said their lower backs ached. These somatic phrases new mothers used to describe their postpartum depression in these cultures have important implications for screening. Screening scales used with mothers in these countries need some items that address these somatic symptoms so that the scale can achieve acceptable levels of sensitivity and specificity.

Developing Middle Range Theory

Qualitative research can represent a rich vein of valuable data for the development of middle range theories. Theoretical frameworks, such as a midrange theory, are essential for designing quantitative studies in a research program. Theoretical coalescence (Morse, in press) is one method that researchers can use to develop a middle range theory. This method involves combining a series of studies on a topic to create a higher, more abstract-level midrange theory. I constructed the middle range theory of Traumatic Childbirth: The Ever-Widening Ripple Effect using Morse's theoretical coalescence (Beck, 2015). The scope of this qualitative theory was increased by formalizing the links among 14 of my studies conducted on traumatic childbirth. The long-term chronic consequences of birth trauma were highlighted not only for mothers in this midrange theory but also for fathers and clinicians present at the traumatic birth. The consequences of a traumatic childbirth can spread out like ripples when a pebble is dropped into a pond (Figure 4.3).

Intervention Studies

When conducting intervention studies, the interplay with qualitative data can provide ideas for studies in a program of research. Qualitative data can help a researcher design an effective intervention. Qualitative data can also help salvage a quantitative intervention.

• **FIGURE 4.3 The Ever-Widening Ripple Effect**
Traumatic Childbirth

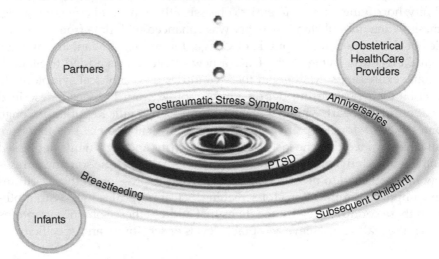

PTSD, posttraumatic stress disorder.
Reprinted with permission from Beck (2015, p. 9).

Morse (2006) asked, "Where do interventions come from?" Vital for developing interventions is qualitative research. Morse listed six broad areas of qualitative research that scientists can use to develop and test interventions:

1. Providing a theoretical foundation for designing effective interventions
2. Providing an approach to identify covert interventions
3. Providing a way to design interventions that are less mechanical in nature
4. Providing a broader scope of practice
5. Providing an expanded definition of an intervention
6. Providing an approach to assess interventions

Back in 1995, Weinholtz, Kacer, and Rocklin published an article entitled, "Salvaging quantitative research with qualitative data." Their abstract read as follows:

> Through presentation of two case studies, this article illustrates just how ambiguous and misleading results from quantitative studies can be if not supplemented by qualitative data. The focus is on the salvaging power of qualitative methods and their ability to ensure some return on an investment that might otherwise be partially or completely lost. (p. 388)

Weinholtz et al. (1995), in their first example of a study of small group instruction of computer applications, illustrated how the use of supplemental qualitative data resulted in insightful interpretation of this research that had reported nonsignificant findings. Their second example involved a study of teaching by university hospital attending physicians. In this study, the qualitative data led the researchers to detect errors in their quantitative data analysis procedures.

Sandelowski (1996) argued against the misconceptions that the relevance of qualitative methods in intervention studies contribute to their lack of use in these quantitative studies. She stressed that "Qualitative methods are especially useful for further describing or exploring subject variation on outcome variables verifying outcomes obtained from standardized instruments, and clarifying and evaluating interventions in their real-life contexts" (p. 359).

With the tremendous interest in mixed methods in the past decade, quantitative researchers are acknowledging the value of adding a qualitative component to their intervention studies. Creswell and Plano Clark (2011) call this type of mixed methods an embedded design. A researcher can embed a qualitative component for several reasons, such as, "to improve recruitment procedures, examine the process of an intervention, or to explain reactions to participation in an experiment" (p. 91).

Internet Qualitative Studies in Research Programs

Qualitative researchers are now beginning to use the Internet to collect data via e-mail, discussion lists, chat rooms, blogs, bulletin board systems, and websites. In the past, the mainstay of qualitative research has been face-to-face interviews. At some point in your program of research, you may want to consider the Internet for data collection. Let us look at some of the advantages and disadvantages of the use of the Internet in qualitative research.

The Internet can be cost-efficient and time saving in interviewing participants compared with face-to-face interviews. In qualitative research, one of the most expensive parts of a budget can be for transcribing interviews. Qualitative data collected over the Internet do not require transcription. The participants have already typed their narratives, so all a researcher needs to do is press the print button. This is such a gift that, to me as a qualitative researcher, it feels like Christmas every time I print out a participant's story. Internet interviews are also time saving since the researcher does not have to schedule a time to meet for a face-to-face interview or travel to interview the participant. Another benefit is that the researcher does not have to worry about considering time zone differences when communicating with study participants. Im and Chee (2003) have termed this advantage asynchronous interaction.

An additional advantage of the Internet in qualitative research is that international representation of study participants is possible. In my research on traumatic childbirth, I have had women participate from countries such as New Zealand, Australia, Canada, and the United Kingdom. The use of the Internet is a valuable approach to sample hidden populations. When data are collected via the Internet, there is a lesser chance of the participants' responses being affected by social desirability and inhibition compared with face-to-face interviews. Also, Internet interviews permit participants time to reflect on their responses to the researcher's questions.

In all my qualitative studies on traumatic childbirth, I have used the Internet to collect mothers' stories. At first, I was leery of how successful this approach would be in obtaining vivid, rich descriptions of mothers' experiences of birth trauma. Prior to this, I had always used face-to-face interviews when conducting my qualitative studies on postpartum depression, and mothers shared their powerful stories with me. How successful would it be to try and repeat this without being in the same room with mothers letting them see my caring? Well, it turned out to be far beyond what I had ever hoped for. I believe that I was able to collect richer data via the Internet than I ever would have in face-to-face interviews. The mothers in my studies would tell me that they would pick away at their stories of their traumatic childbirth a little bit at a time. They would save their story on their computer and go back to it at a later date to continue on with it. There was only so much the women could handle at one time reliving their birth trauma. If I had interviewed these women face-to-face, I believe I would not have obtained the powerful, detailed narratives these mothers were able to send me via the Internet. In a 1-hour face-to-face interview, there would have been only so much the mothers could have handled sharing with me.

What are some of the limitations of using the Internet for qualitative data collection? In qualitative research, it is the researcher who is the instrument for data collection, not reliable and valid questionnaires. Strickland et al. (2003) have cautioned that successful qualitative data collection via the Internet is heavily dependent on the researcher's interview skill within the constraints of the Internet. Cotton (2003) stressed how critical it is for researchers to be "caring, holistic, and culturally sensitive" (p. 317).

Another limitation is that recruiting participants is limited to individuals with computer skills and access to the Internet. Also, because you are not interviewing participants face-to-face, the researcher is unable to observe nonverbal cues or changes in voice intonations. A low response rate to online data collection is another potential limitation that qualitative researchers need to consider. Hamilton and Bowers (2006) suggest that a response rate be computed for Internet samples. In my qualitative Internet studies on traumatic childbirth, I have done this calculation. Response rates are based on the number of individuals who initially contact the researcher for information on the qualitative study and go on to actually participate in the study. Here is an excerpt from my study on the impact of birth trauma on breastfeeding:

> In the current study 129 women initially responded to the Internet recruitment notice and requested more detailed information about the research. Out of these 129 women, 75 participated in the study, for a 58% response rate. (Beck & Watson, 2008, p. 230)

In all my phenomenological studies on traumatic childbirth, I have used e-mail to collect my data. I purposely chose this Internet method because I wanted to have the ability to communicate individually with my participants even if I could not do that in person face-to-face. The most time-consuming part of collecting data this way was crafting my individual e-mail responses to the mothers. I wanted to make sure I conveyed my concern and caring for them and my absolute gratitude to them for sharing such personal stories with me, a stranger. I wanted to develop a rapport and begin a trusting relationship. In my initial response to potential participants, I promised to honor their words to the best of my ability to educate health care providers about birth trauma and its resulting posttraumatic stress disorder.

In 2005, I conducted a qualitative secondary data analysis to identify the repetitive themes of the benefits mothers had received by participating in my birth trauma study over the Internet. Content analysis revealed seven themes (Beck, 2005):

- Experienced caring by being listened to and acknowledged
- Sense of belonging
- Making sense of it all
- Letting go of details about their birth trauma
- Being empowered
- Women helping women
- Providing a voice

I believe the participants experienced these benefits due to the care I took in crafting my responses to them in my e-mails.

There are endless possibilities for using different research designs in a research program. With my traumatic childbirth research, I have been focusing on qualitative studies where all the data are collected via the Internet. A variation of this that a researcher may decide to use is a data source triangulation including both online and offline collection of qualitative data. Orgad (2009) addressed the importance of researchers considering both online and offline data in a qualitative study. Hine (2000) suggested that studying participants in their offline environments can be a valuable way to contextualize data obtained on the Internet, and also that it can add authenticity to those online results. I used data source triangulation of online and offline interviews in my research study with mothers whose children suffered obstetric brachial plexus injuries as a result of shoulder dystocia births (Beck, 2009). In this phenomenological study, 11 mothers participated in my study via the Internet, and 12 women were interviewed face-to-face by me. Use of both data sources provided an opportunity to ascertain that a consistent portrayal of the phenomenon emerged.

MIXED METHODS AS AN OPTION IN RESEARCH PROGRAMS

Mayring (2007) described mixed methods research as "a new star in the social science sky" (p. 1). Mixed methods research has also been called the "third research paradigm" (Johnson & Onwuegbuzie, 2004, p. 15). The first paradigm is quantitative research, and the second is qualitative research. In the past 10 years, interest in mixed methods has increased tremendously. In mixed methods, the researcher

- Collects and analyzes persuasively and rigorously both qualitative and quantitative data (based on research questions)
- Mixes (or integrates or links) the two forms of data concurrently by combining them (or merging them), sequentially by having one build on the other, or embedding one within the other
- Gives priority to one or to both forms of data (in terms of what the research emphasizes)
- Uses these procedures in a single study or in multiple phases of a program of study
- Frames these procedures within philosophical worldviews and theoretical lenses, and
- Combines the procedures into specific research designs that direct the plan for conducting the study. (Creswell & Plano Clark, 2011, p. 5)

When is it appropriate for a researcher to use a mixed methods approach in a program of research? What types of research problems fit mixed methods inquiry? When traditional approaches of data collection using one method are not adequate for answering complex research questions, a "plurality of methodological approaches and philosophical perspectives" may be needed (Hesse-Biber & Johnson, 2013, p. 103). Creswell and Plano Clark (2011) identified six situations that would warrant designing a mixed methods study:

1. A need exists because one data source is insufficient
2. A need exists to explain initial results of a study
3. A need exists to generalize exploratory results
4. A need exists to enhance understanding of a study with a second method
5. A need exists to use a theoretical perspective
6. A need exists to understand a research objective by multiple research phases

Once a researcher decides that a mixed methods approach is the most appropriate path to take for the next study in a program of research, a choice needs to be made concerning a specific design that best fits the research problem. Creswell and Plano Clark (2011) identified 15 different typologies of mixed methods designs. Researchers need to review carefully these typologies and choose the one that is the best fit for their research questions. For example, Morse and Niehaus (2009), in their typology, do not include a mixed methods design when both the quantitative and qualitative strands are equal. In their typology, one of the strands needs to be the driving force with priority over the other strand. Creswell and Plano Clark, however, do have a mixed methods design in their typology, where both the quantitative and the qualitative strands are equal.

The choice of which mixed methods design to use rests on four key decisions (Creswell & Plano Clark, 2011). The first is the level of interaction between the quantitative and the qualitative strands. This refers to the degree to which the two strands are kept independent or interact with each other. Will the two strands be kept separate until the final interpretation or mixed before that? The second key decision involves determining the priority of the quantitative and qualitative strands. Will the two strands have equal priority? Will the quantitative strand have priority, or will the qualitative strand have priority? Next to be decided is the timing of the two strands. Timing refers to the order in which the findings from the two data sets are used within the study. Timing can be concurrent, sequential, or multiphase combination (Creswell & Plano Clark, 2011). Concurrent timing refers to implementing both the quantitative and the qualitative strands during a single phase of the study. In sequential timing, the two strands are implemented in two separate phases where data collection and analysis of one type of data occur after data collection and analysis of the other. It is the researcher's choice which type of data (quantitative or qualitative) will be collected and analyzed first. Multiphase combination timing refers to implementing multiple phases in a program of research that includes concurrent and/or sequential timing. The fourth and final key decision revolves around the procedures for mixing the quantitative and qualitative strands. The point in the mixed methods study where the two strands are mixed is called the point of interface (Morse & Niehaus, 2009). Mixing can occur during data collection, data analysis, or during the final step of interpretation of the two analyzed data sets.

As previously stated, there are 15 varieties of typologies of mixed methods designs. In this chapter, I will concentrate on Creswell and Plano Clark's typology as one illustration (Figure 4.4). They proposed six types of mixed methods designs:

1. Concurrent parallel design: In this design, concurrent timing, equal priority of methods, independent strands during analysis, and mixing at interpretation occur.

• **FIGURE 4.4** Prototypical Versions of the Six Major Mixed Methods Research Designs: (a) the Convergent Parallel Design; (b) the Explanatory Sequential Design; (c) the Exploratory Sequential Design; (d) the Embedded Design; (e) the Transformative Design; and (f) the Multiphase Design

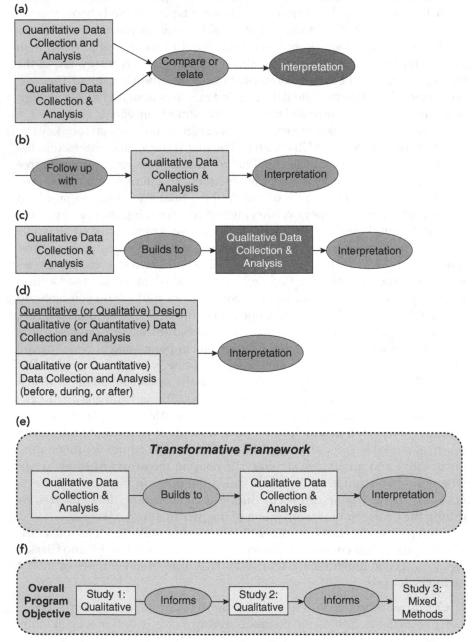

Reprinted with permission from Creswell and Plano Clark (2011, pp. 69–70).

2. Explanatory sequential design: Here, the priority is the quantitative strand. Data collection and analysis of quantitative data are done first. The second phase is the qualitative phase, where the researcher uses the qualitative data to explain the quantitative results of the first phase.
3. Exploratory sequential design: The qualitative strand is given priority, so the first phase involves data collection of qualitative data. In the second phase, quantitative data are used to test or generalize the qualitative results.
4. Embedded design: This design involves adding a supplemental strand to improve the overall design. A researcher may add a quantitative strand within a qualitative design or add a qualitative strand within a quantitative design.
5. Transformative design: Here, a mixed methods design is framed within a transformative theoretical framework that addresses the needs of a vulnerable population in order to make change.
6. Mulitphase design: This design involves the combination of concurrent and/or sequential collection of qualitative and quantitative data sets over multiple phases of a research program.

Morse (2012) argued for addition of mixed methods designs when both strands are qualitative. Simultaneous and sequential qualitative mixed methods designs are options for researchers in their program of research. In Morse's typology of mixed methods, there is always a core component and a supplementary component. In a QUAL-qual design, the core component is a complete method such as phenomenology, ethnography, or grounded theory. The supplementary component is a research strategy used in other qualitative methods such as a specific interviewing type or observational technique. A supplementary component is not a complete method:

> The supplemental component may be paced simultaneously or sequentially. The pacing and the type of research strategy are so chosen as to best enable the research question to be answered:
>
> 1. More fully or more comprehensively (with broader scope or increased depth), therefore making the research richer and more useful, or
>
> 2. To obtain another perspective, using a different data type (such as observational data to conduct a core project that uses interviews), or
>
> 3. To obtain data from a different level of analysis or abstraction—for instance, the core project may use broadly categorized participant observational data, and the supplementary component may use videotaped data that are micro analyzed, thereby adding detail so that the project better answers the research question, and

4. To provide information that may have been inaccessible or un-
available when using one method alone or to answer a sub-
question that cannot be answered within the core component
(and therefore moves the research program along).

5. In addition, designs embodying a sequential supplemental qualitative component are used: to answer minor questions that have
emerged from the core project, or to move the project toward
implementation—for instance, to develop an assessment guide
from a grounded theory core component. (Morse, 2012, p. 555)

Researchers who are considering a mixed methods study in their program
of research need to be aware of some challenges in using mixed methods.
The first is the question of skills. Does the researcher have the necessary basic skills in both quantitative and qualitative methods? Next, the researcher
needs to consider whether a mixed methods study is feasible given time
and resources. Does the researcher have enough time for data collection and
analysis of two types of data? Does the researcher have enough resources to
collect and analyze both quantitative and qualitative data sets? Lastly, does
the researcher have personnel available with the skills for both data sets?

In conducting mixed methods research, one needs to have a range of
skills. Morgan (2014) proposed three approaches to build that expertise in
integrating quantitative and qualitative methods: individual mastery, teamwork, and boundary spanning. In individual mastery, one person has a level
of mastery for both quantitative and qualitative skills. Morgan states that it
is unlikely that one researcher has high-level skills in each method. In teamwork, a minimum level of any additional preparation is needed on the part of
the researchers since the existing skills within the team can be used. In boundary spanning, a researcher requires prior preparation in one of the methods
and also close familiarity with the other method. In Table 4.5, Morgan (2014)
describes the characteristics of teamwork in mixed methods research.

Another scar to my soul: Secondary traumatic stress in labor and delivery nurses (Beck & Gable, 2012) is an example of a mixed methods study
from my program of research. What led me to take the untrodden path of conducting a mixed methods study when I had never used this design method
before? For the prior 10 years, I had been investigating mothers' experiences
of traumatic childbirth using descriptive phenomenology as the method of
choice. Often, when presenting the findings of these qualitative studies at conferences, obstetric nurses in the audience would say that I should study them
too. The nurses said they were just as traumatized as the mothers when birth
trauma occurs. So I did a literature search and found the concept of secondary
traumatic stress. Figley (1995) defined secondary traumatic stress as "the natural consequent behaviors and emotions resulting from knowledge about a
traumatizing event experienced by a significant other. This stress results from

• **TABLE 4.5 Characteristics of Teamwork in Mixed Methods Research**

Team Culture	
Shared vocabulary	Team members are "bilingual" with regard to each other's typical procedures and specific jargon.
Mutual respect	Team members understand the value of each other's contributions and value what the others can offer.
Mutual understanding	Team members understand the "why" behind each other's methods and research designs.
Division of Labor	
Multidisciplinary	Qualitative and quantitative researchers each possess separate strengths that operate in parallel.
Interdisciplinary	Qualitative and quantitative researchers work together to make use of each other's strengths.
Transdisciplinary	Qualitative and quantitative researchers share their strengths in ways that affect how both methods operate.
Leadership	
Communication	Leader(s) encourage exchanges that allow both qualitative and quantitative researchers to follow each other's activities.
Coordination	Leader(s) bring together qualitative and quantitative researchers to discuss each other's decisions.
Collaboration	Leader(s) actively unite qualitative and quantitative researchers for shared decision making.

Reprinted with permission from Morgan (2014, p. 220).

helping or wanting to help a traumatized or suffering person" (p. 10). Figley warned health care providers of possible harmful effects of secondary exposure to traumatic events of patients to whom they are providing care. These harmful effects are similar to those of posttraumatic stress disorder.

Three research questions I wanted to investigate in my first mixed methods study were:

1. What are the prevalence and severity of secondary traumatic stress in labor and delivery nurses due to exposure to traumatic childbirth?
2. What are the experiences of labor and delivery nurses who are present at traumatic births?
3. How do the qualitative experiences of labor and delivery nurses inform the quantitative results of the Secondary Traumatic Stress Scale (STSS; Bride, Robinson, Yegidis, & Figley, 2004)?

In deciding on which mixed methods design I would use for my study on secondary traumatic stress in labor and delivery nurses, I believed that neither the qualitative nor the quantitative strand would have priority, so I chose Creswell and Plano Clark's (2011) convergent parallel design. A random sample of 464 labor and delivery nurses who were members of the Association of Women's Health, Obstetric, and Neonatal Nurses (AWHONN) was obtained. Nurses first completed the STSS and next were asked to describe in depth their experiences of being present at traumatic childbirths. Quantitative data analysis revealed 35% of the sample reported moderate to severe levels of secondary traumatic stress. From the qualitative data analysis six themes emerged: "(1) Magnifying the exposure to traumatic births, (2) Struggling to maintain a professional role while with traumatized patients, (3) Agonizing over what should have been, (4) Mitigating the aftermath of exposure to traumatic births, (5) Haunted by secondary traumatic stress symptoms, and (6) Considering forgoing careers in labor and delivery to survive" (Beck & Gable, 2012, p. 747).

As a certified nurse-midwife (CNM) myself, I was interested in investigating the prevalence of second traumatic stress in CNMs. How did the prevalence rate of secondary traumatic stress in CNMs compare with that of the labor and delivery nurses in my first mixed methods study? Using Survey Monkey, 473 CNMs completed the STSS and then were asked to describe their experiences attending traumatic births (Beck, LoGiudice, & Gable, 2015) In this sample 42% of the CNMs reported moderate to severe levels of secondary traumatic stress. Six themes emerged from this qualitative strand of the mixed methods study:

1. Protecting my patients: Agonizing sense of powerlessness and helplessness
2. Wreaking havoc: Trio of posttraumatic stress symptoms
3. Circling the wagons: It takes a team to provide support...or not
4. Litigation: Nowhere to go to unburden our souls
5. Shaken belief in the birth process: Impacting midwifery practice
6. Moving on: Where do I go from here?

REFERENCES

Beck, A. T., Steer, R. A., & Brown, G. K. (1996). *BDI-II manual*. San Antonio, TX: The Psychological Corporation.
Beck, C. T. (1992). The lived experience of postpartum depression: A phenomenological study. *Nursing Research, 41,* 166–170.
Beck, C. T. (1993). Teetering on the edge: A substantive theory of postpartum depression. *Nursing Research, 42,* 42–48.
Beck, C. T. (1996). Postpartum depressed mothers' experiences interacting with their children. *Nursing Research, 45,* 98–104.
Beck, C. T. (2005). Benefits of participating in Internet interviews: Women helping women. *Qualitative Health Research, 15* (3), 411–422.

Beck, C. T. (2007). Exemplar: Teetering on the edge: A continually emerging theory of postpartum depression. In P. L. Munhall (Ed.), *Nursing research: A qualitative perspective* (pp. 273–292). Sudbury, MA: Jones & Bartlett.

Beck, C. T. (2009). The arm: There is no escaping the reality for mothers of children with obstetric brachial plexus injuries. *Nursing Research, 58,* 237–245.

Beck, C. T. (2012). Exemplar: Teetering on the edge: A second grounded theory modification. In P. L. Munhall (Ed.), *Nursing research: A qualitative perspective* (pp. 257–284). Sudbury, MA: Jones & Bartlett.

Beck, C. T. (2013). The obstetric nightmare of shoulder dystocia: A tale from two perspectives. *MCN: The American Journal of Maternal Child Nursing, 38*(1), 34–40.

Beck, C. T. (2015). Middle range theory of traumatic childbirth: The ever-widening ripple effect. *Global Qualitative Nursing Research, 2,* 1–13. doi:10.1177/23333936 15575313

Beck, C. T., & Gable, R. K. (2000). Postpartum Depression Screening Scale: Development and psychometric testing. *Nursing Research, 49,* 272–282.

Beck, C. T., & Gable, R. K. (2001a). Ensuring content validity: An illustration of the process. *Journal of Nursing Measurement, 9*(2), 201–215.

Beck, C. T. & Gable, R. K. (2001b). Further validation of the Postpartum Depression Screening Scale. *Nursing Research, 50,* 155–164.

Beck, C. T., & Gable, R. K. (2001c). Comparative analysis of the performance of the Postpartum Depression Screening Scale with two other depression instruments. *Nursing Research, 50,* 242–250.

Beck, C. T., & Gable, R. K. (2002). *Postpartum Depression Screening Scale manual.* Los Angeles, CA: Western Psychological Services.

Beck, C. T., & Gable, R.K. (2012). A mixed methods study: Secondary traumatic stress in labor and delivery nurses. *Journal of Obstetric, Gynecologic, and Neonatal Nursing, 41,* 747–760.

Beck, C. T., LoGiudice, J., & Gable, R. K. (2015). Shaken belief in the birth process: A mixed methods study of secondary traumatic stress in certified nurse-midwives. *Journal of Midwifery & Women's Health, 60,* 16–23.

Beck, C. T., & Watson, S. (2008). Impact of birth trauma on breast-feeding: A tale of two pathways. *Nursing Research, 57*(4), 228–236.

Bride, B. E., Robinson, M. M., Yegidis, B., & Figley, C. R. (2004). Development and validation of the Secondary Traumatic Stress Scale. *Research on Social Work Practice, 14,* 27–35.

Cantilino, A., Carvalho, J. A., Maia, A., Albuquerque, C., Cantilino, G., & Sougey, E. B. (2007). Translation, validation and cultural aspects of Postpartum Depression Screening Scale in Brazilian Portuguese. *Transcultural Psychiatry, 44*(4), 672–684.

Clarke, P. J. (2008). Validation of two postpartum depression screening scales with a sample of First Nations and Métis women. *Canadian Journal of Nursing Research, 40* (1), 113–125.

Cotton, A. H. (2003). The discursive field of Web-based health research: Implications for nursing research in cyberspace. *Advances in Nursing Science, 26,* 307–319.

Cox, J. L., Holden, J. M., & Sagovsky, R. (1987). Detection of postnatal depression: Development of the 10-item Edinburgh Postnatal Depression Scale. *British Journal of Psychiatry, 150,* 782–786.

Creswell, J. W., & Plano Clark, V. L. (2011). *Designing and conducting mixed methods research*. Los Angeles, CA: SAGE.

Figley, C. R. (1995). Compassion fatigue: Toward a new understanding of the costs of caring. In B. H. Stamm (Ed.), *Secondary traumatic stress: Self-care uses for clinicians, researchers, and educators* (pp. 3–28). Lutherville, MD: Sidran Press.

Fleury, J. (1993). Preserving qualitative meaning in instrument development. *Journal of Nursing Measurement, 1*, 135–144.

Gable, R. K., & Wolf, M. (1993). *Instrument development in the affective domain*. Norwell, MA: Kluwer Academic.

Glaser, B. G. (1998). *Doing grounded theory: Issues and discussions*. Mill Valley, CA: Sociology Press.

Glaser, B. G. (2001). *The grounded theory perspective: Conceptualization contrasted with description*. Mill Valley, CA: Sociology Press.

Glaser, B. G., & Strauss, A. L. (1967). *The discovery of grounded theory*. New York: Aldine de Gruyter.

Hall, J. M. (2000). Women survivors of childhood abuse: The impact of traumatic stress on education and work. *Issues in Mental Health Nursing, 21*, 443–471.

Hamilton, R. J., & Bowers, B. J. (2006). Internet recruitment and email interviews in qualitative studies. *Qualitative Health Research, 16* (6), 821–835.

Hesse-Biber, S., & Johnson, R. B. (2013). Coming at things differently: Future directions of possible engagement with mixed methods research. *Journal of Mixed Methods Research, 7*, 103–109.

Hinds, P. S., Vogel, R. J., & Clarke-Steffen, L. (1997). The possibilities and pitfalls of doing a secondary analysis of a qualitative data set. *Qualitative Health Research, 7* (3), 408–424.

Hine, C. (2000). *Virtual ethnography*. London, UK: SAGE.

Im, E. O., & Chee, W. (2003). Issues in Internet research. *Nursing Outlook, 51*, 6–12.

Imle, M., & Atwood, J. (1988). Retaining qualitative validity while gaining quantitative reliability and validity: Development of the Transition to Parenthood Concerns Scale. *Advances in Nursing Science, 11*, 61–75.

Johnson, R. B., & Onwuegbuzie, A. J. (2004). Mixed methods research: A research paradigm whose time has come. *Educational Researcher, 33* (7), 14–26.

Karacam, Z., & Kitis, Y. (2008). The Postpartum Depression Screening Scale: Its reliability and validity for the Turkish population. *Turkish Journal of Psychiatry, 19*(2), 1–10.

Kossakowska, K. (2012). A Polish adaptation and psychometric evaluation of the Postpartum Depression Screening Scale (PDSS) for diagnosing symptoms and signs of postnatal depression. *Postepy Psychiatrii i Neurologii, 21* (2), 123–129.

Krippendorff, K. (2013). *Content analysis: An introduction to its methodology*. Thousand Oaks, CA: SAGE.

Lara, M. A., Navarrete, L., Navarro, C., & Le, H. N. (2013). Evaluation of the psychometric measures for the Postpartum Depression Screening Scale-Spanish version for Mexican women. *Journal of Transcultural Nursing, 24* (4), 378–386.

Li, L., Liu, F., Zhang, H., Wang, L., & Wiaofang, C. (2011). Chinese version of the Postpartum Depression Screening Scale: Translation and validation. *Nursing Research, 60* (4), 231–239.

Maia, B. R., Marques, M., Bos, S., Pereira, A. T., Soares, M. J., Valente, J., . . . Azevedo, M. H. (2011). Epidemiology of perinatal depression in Portugal: Categorical and dimensional approach. *Acta Medica Portuguesa, 24*(Suppl. 2), 443–448.

Mayring, P. (2007). Introduction: Arguments for mixed methodology. In P. Mayring, G. L. Huber, L. Gurtler, & M. Kiegelmann (Eds.), *Mixed methodology in psychological research* (pp. 1–4). Rotterdam/Taipei: Sense.

McCoach, B. D., Gable, R. K., & Madura, J. P. (2013). *Instrument development in the affective domain: School and corporate applications.* New York, NY: Springer.

Morgan, D. L. (2014*). Integrating qualitative and quantitative methods: A pragmatic approach.* Los Angeles, CA: SAGE.

Morse, J. M. (2006). The scope of qualitatively derived clinical interventions. *Qualitative Health Research, 16* (5), 591–593.

Morse, J. M. (2012). Simultaneous and sequential qualitative mixed-methods designs. In P. L. Munhall (Ed.), *Nursing research: A qualitative perspective* (pp. 553–569). Sudbury, MA: Jones & Bartlett Learning.

Morse, J. M. (in press). *Analyzing and constructing the conceptual and theoretical foundations of nursing.* Philadelphia, PA: F.A. Davis.

Morse, J. M., & Niehaus, L. (2009). *Mixed methods design: Principles and procedures.* Walnut Creek, CA: Left Coast Press.

Morse, J. M., & Pooler, C. (2002). Patient-family-nurse interactions in the trauma-resuscitation room. *American Journal of Critical Care, 11*(3), 240–249.

Orgad, S. (2009). How can researchers make sense of the issues involved in collecting and interpreting online and offline data? In A. N. Markham & N. K. Baym (Eds.), *Internet inquiry: Conversations about method* (pp. 33–60). Los Angeles, CA: SAGE.

Pereira, A. T., Bos, S., Marques, M., Maia, B. R., Soares, M. J., Valente, J. . . . Azevedo, M. H. (2010). The Portuguese version of the Postpartum Depression Screening Scale. *Journal of Psychosomatic Obstetrics & Gynecology, 31*(2), 90–100.

Pereira, A. T., Bos, S., Marques, M., Maia, B., Soares, M. J., Valente, J., . . . Macedo, A. (2013). Short form of the Postpartum Depression Screening Scale: As accurate as the original form. *Archives of Women's Mental Health, 16, 67–77.*

Quelopana, A. M. (2012). Violence against women and postpartum depression: The experience of Chilean women. *Women & Health, 52,* 437–453.

Quelopana, A. M., & Champion, J. D. (2010). Validation of the Postpartum Depression Screening Scale-Spanish Version in women from Arica, Chile. *Ciencia y Enfermeria, 16*(1), 37–47.

Quelopana, A. M., Champion, J. D., & Reyes-Rubilar, T. (2011). Factors associated with postpartum depression in Chilean women. *Health Care for Women International, 32,* 939–949.

Sandelowski, M. (1996). Using qualitative methods in intervention studies. *Research in Nursing & Health, 19,* 359–364.

Sandelowski, M. J. (1997a). Programmatic qualitative research: Or, appreciating the importance of gas station pumps. In J. M. Morse (Ed.), *Completing a qualitative project: Details and dialogue* (pp. 211–225). Thousand Oaks, CA: SAGE.

Sandelowski, M. (1997b). "To be of use": Enhancing the utility of qualitative research. *Nursing Outlook, 45*(3), 125–132.

Sharrock, W. W., & Anderson, D. C. (1979). Directional hospital signs as sociological data. *Information Design Journal, 1*, 81–94.

Strickland, O. L., Moloney, M. F., Dietrich, A. S., Myerburg, S., Cotsonis, G. A., & Johnson, R. V. (2003). Measurement issues related to data collection on the World Wide Web. *Advances in Nursing Science, 26*(4), 246–256.

Tate, J. A., Dabbs, A. D., Hoffman, L. A., Milbrandt, E., & Happ, M. B. (2012). Anxiety and agitation in mechanically ventilated patients. *Qualitative Health Research, 22*(2), 157–173.

Thorne, S. (2013). Secondary qualitative data analysis. In C. T. Beck (Ed.), *Routledge international handbook of qualitative nursing research* (pp. 393–404). New York, NY: Routledge.

Tilden, V. P., Nelson, C. A., & May, B. A. (1990). Use of qualitative methods to enhance content validity. *Nursing Research, 39*(3), 172–175.

Van Manen, M. (1990). *Researching lived experience: Human science for an action sensitive pedagogy.* New York, NY: Albany State University of New York Press.

Vittayanont, A., Liabsuetrakul, T., & Pitanupong, J. (2006). Development of the Post-partum Depression Screening Scale (PDSS): A Thai version for screening post-partum depression. *Journal of the Medical Association of Thailand, 89*(1), 1–7.

Weinholtz, D., Kacer, B., & Rocklin, T. (1995). Salvaging quantitative research with qualitative data. *Qualitative Health Research, 5*(3), 388–397.

Zubaran, C., Foresti, K., Schmacher, M. V., Amoretti, A. L., Miller, C., Thorell, M. R., . . . Madi, J. M. (2009). Validation of a screening instrument for postpartum depression in Southern Brazil. *Journal of Psychometric Obstetrics & Gynecology, 30*(4), 244–254.

Zubaran, C., & Foresti, K. (2011). Investigating quality of life and depressive symptoms in the postpartum period. *Women and Birth, 24*, 10–16.

Zubaran, C., & Foresti, K. (2013). The correlation between breastfeeding, self-efficacy and maternal postpartum depression in southern Brazil. *Sexual & Reproductive Healthcare, 4*, 9–15.

Zubaran, C., Foresti, K., Schmacher, M. V., Amoretti, A. L., Miller, C., Thorell, M. R., & Müller, L. C. (2010a). Correlation between postpartum depression and health sta-tus. *Maternal Child Health Journal, 14*, 751–757.

Zubaran, C., Foresti, K., Schmacher, M. V., Amoretti, A. L., Miller, C., Thorell, M. R., & Müller, L. C. (2010b). The Portuguese version of the Postpartum Depression Screening Scale-Short Form. *Journal of Obstetrics and Gynaecology Research, 36*(5), 950–957.

Sustaining a Program of Research

Remember when life's path is steep to keep your
mind even.

—*Horace*

CHARACTERISTICS OF A SUCCESSFUL PROGRAM OF RESEARCH AND STEPS TO ACHIEVE IT

Reflecting on their research program, Wuest and Hodgins (2011) shared that "programs of research often have very humble beginnings in isolated studies. The thread that binds studies together becomes apparent over time and through reflection. . . . Synthesizing a program of research requires attention to the conceptual findings and methodological approaches in the context of pragmatic influences on the program's evolution" (p. 151).

Holzemer (2009) stated that "Building a program of research is not really a linear process, but more an iterative process where you begin again and begin again. It is a repetitive process, where you think about your area of interest differently. You might see knowledge build incrementally or maybe there are quantum leaps of change in your understanding. The process itself is somewhat unpredictable" (p. 2). Holzemer (2009) identified the following essential characteristics of a good research program: feasible, interesting, novel, ethical, and relevant. His eight steps to building a research trajectory include:

1. Know your passion
2. Ensure high public health significance
3. Know the literature in your field
4. Understand clinical practice in your area
5. Use the outcomes model to think about your program of research

6. Nurture interdisciplinary colleagues
7. Publish-building from study to study
8. Have fun along the journey (p. 5)

Being successful in developing a valuable program of research involves a step-by-step progression whereby nurse scientists systematically build expertise in their specific research area. Figure 5.1 is a research trajectory for building a program of research that consists of a systematically planned series of interrelated and iterative steps, outlined by Gitlin and Lyons (2008, p. 18), that can move a person from novice, to intermediate, to advanced, and to expert.

Each level of expertise in Gitlin and Lyon's systematic approach consists of three fundamental activities: presentations at professional conferences, publishing in professional journals, and conducting research.

Securing external funding through grants is critical, especially in quantitative and mixed methods studies. In this day and age of limited and unpredictable funding streams, competition is fierce. The National Institutes of Health (NIH), for example, offers career awards, known as the K series, that can provide a researcher with protected time to carry out training and research activities. The K series has different categories of career awards that researchers can apply for, depending on the stage they are at in their program of research: postdoctoral training, midcareer, or established investigators. The criteria for successfully securing a K award include the likelihood that the investigator will sustain a strong research trajectory. Taken into consideration are the following: the researcher, career plan for development, research plan, mentors, collaborators, and the environment and commitment of the institution where the investigator is employed.

NIH also offers research grants for investigators. Listed are some of the frequently used research grant programs:

- R01 NIH research project grant program
- R03 NIH small grant program
- R13 NIH support for conferences and scientific meetings
- R15 NIH academic research enhancement award (AREA)
- R21 NIH exploratory/developmental research grant award
- R34 NIH clinical trial planning grant program

Grantsmanship is one aspect of a sustained program of research that relies on perseverance. Investigators may have to resubmit their grant proposals multiple times, based on the reviewers' feedback. Investigators should also consider private foundations as a source of research funding, as I did in my research trajectory. The Patrick and Catherine Weldon Donaghue Medical Research Foundation in West Hartford, Connecticut, funded three of my grants. The first grant was to develop and psychometrically test my Postpartum Depression Screening Scale (PDSS). The second grant was to translate the PDSS into Spanish and test its psychometrics. The third grant allowed me

• FIGURE 5.1 Research Trajectory From Novice to Expert

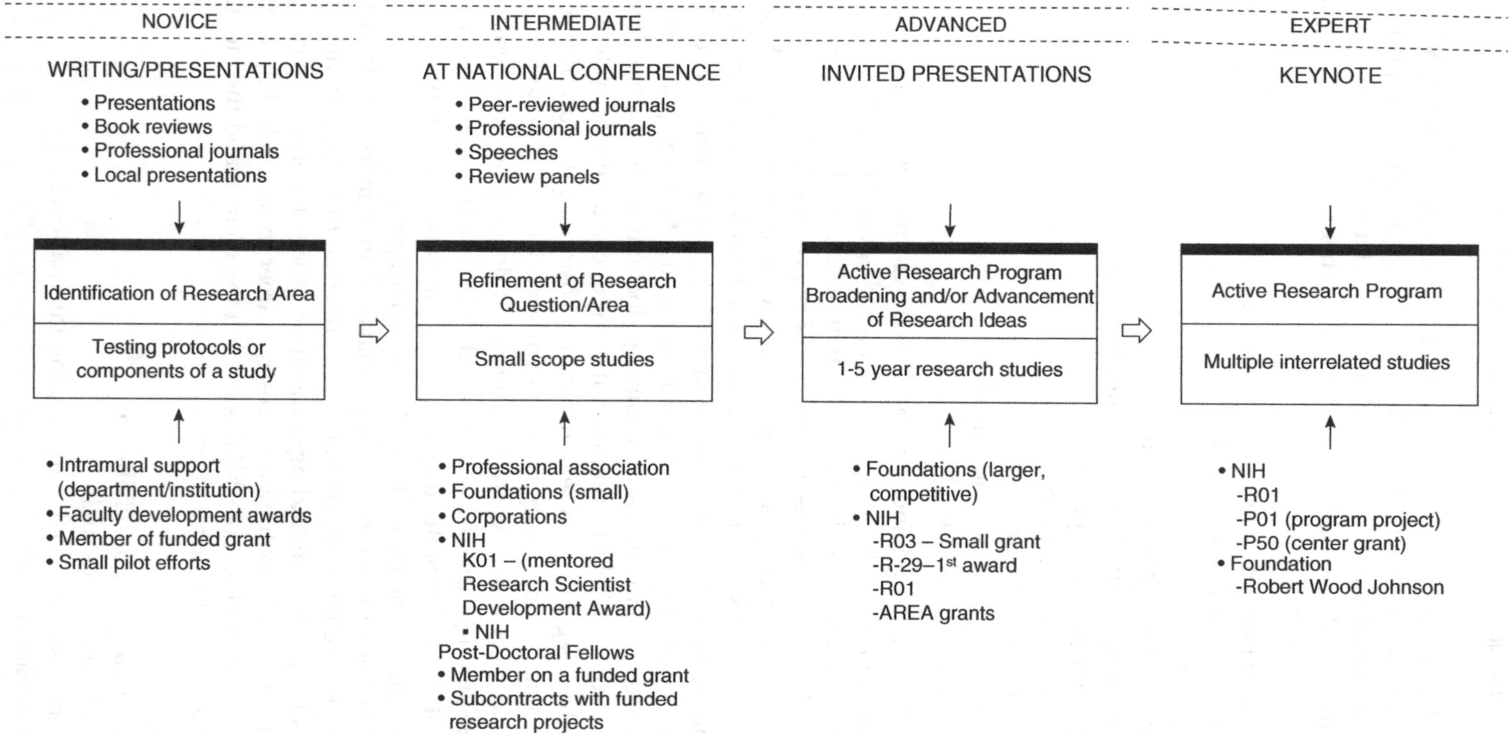

NOVICE	INTERMEDIATE	ADVANCED	EXPERT
WRITING/PRESENTATIONS	AT NATIONAL CONFERENCE	INVITED PRESENTATIONS	KEYNOTE

WRITING/PRESENTATIONS
• Presentations
• Book reviews
• Professional journals
• Local presentations

AT NATIONAL CONFERENCE
• Peer-reviewed journals
• Professional journals
• Speeches
• Review panels

INVITED PRESENTATIONS

KEYNOTE

Identification of Research Area

Testing protocols or components of a study

Refinement of Research Question/Area

Small scope studies

Active Research Program Broadening and/or Advancement of Research Ideas

1-5 year research studies

Active Research Program

Multiple interrelated studies

• Intramural support (department/institution)
• Faculty development awards
• Member of funded grant
• Small pilot efforts

• Professional association
• Foundations (small)
• Corporations
• NIH
  K01 – (mentored Research Scientist Development Award)
  • NIH
  Post-Doctoral Fellows
• Member on a funded grant
• Subcontracts with funded research projects

• Foundations (larger, competitive)
• NIH
  -R03 – Small grant
  -R-29–1st award
  -R01
  -AREA grants

• NIH
  -R01
  -P01 (program project)
  -P50 (center grant)
• Foundation
  -Robert Wood Johnson

Reprinted with permission from Gitlin and Lyons (2008, p. 18).

to conduct a double-blind randomized control trial looking at the impact of a diet enriched in docosahexaenoic acid (DHA) during pregnancy on postpartum depressive symptoms over the first 6 months after birth.

Whittemore (2007) identified the following as her top 10 tips for beginning a research trajectory:

1. Be strategic in planning a program of research
2. Explore postdoctoral opportunities
3. Seek a mentor
4. Seek a research-intensive environment
5. Seek research opportunities and responsibilities
6. Develop grant-writing expertise
7. Talk to others about your ideas
8. Learn about funding opportunities
9. Extend your work and get your ideas out
10. Cultivate several lines of inquiry

Whittemore (2007) reminds us to "remember you are seeking to develop a program of research, not a solitary research study" (p. 237).

In order to successfully launch a research career, faculty mentorship is critical. Conn (2004) stressed the importance of choosing a doctoral program that has experienced faculty advisors who have successful research programs. These research-savvy faculty advisors can be role models to doctoral students who are exposed to these successful research trajectories. Several of these researchers can lead informal seminars on how to develop a research program. Seminars can focus on questioning doctoral students about their subsequent studies to help to reinforce the value of sustained, systematic research as they begin their research careers. Postdoctoral education provides an invaluable opportunity for young nurse scientists to hone their research skills and get more expert mentorship in developing their research programs. Beginning nurse researchers need to be aware that even after the completion of a postdoctorate, they need to be lifelong learners of new research approaches as their trajectories take different paths.

Toto (2008) described three elements that need to be in focus to launch a successful career in clinical research: finding protected time, mentorship, and practical tips for publishing findings. The importance of mentorship cannot be stressed enough in launching a successful career in research. Toto (2008) identified the roles and responsibilities of both the mentor and the mentee. The following pertain to the mentor:

- Inspiration
- Intellectual input/critique/challenge
- Protection of time for research
- Recognition—local, regional, national, and international
- Academic advancement

- Funding
- Success in publication and in promotion and finding a position (Toto, 2008, p. 844)

The mentee's roles and responsibilities are as follows:

- Self-awareness
- Being open with mentor about career plans, needs, and wants
- Preparing before meeting with the mentor
- Setting expectations and reviewing progress regularly
- Being fierce about your work and persevering
- Exercising discipline and perseverance
- Staying focused on research questions
- Knowing strengths and limitations (Toto, 2008, p. 844)

Barriers that need to be overcome in order to achieve a successful research career trajectory include:

- Lack of time/workload
- Lack of availability of resources
- Lack of systematic mentoring
- Lack of institutional support
- Lack of a research culture in an institution (Gitlin & Lyons, 2008, p. 29)

Researchers often cite lack of time as the reason for not developing a systematic program of research. Time management strategies are critical to ensure research productivity and to deal with the competing demands, interruptions, and distractions that researchers have to grapple with while trying to maintain a successful research trajectory. Time management is defined as "behaviours that aim at achieving an effective use of time while performing certain goal-directed activities" (Claessens, Van Eerde, Rutte, & Roe, 2007, p. 262). Claessens and colleagues formulated this definition to emphasize that time should be used not as an end in itself or in isolation, but effectively in pursuit of a goal-directed activity. Claessens et al. (2007) identified three strategies for achieving time management:

1. Time assessment behaviors that focus on a person's being aware of the present, past, and future. Self-awareness of one's use of time can help to facilitate accepting tasks and responsibilities that can fit within a person's capabilities.
2. Planning behaviors that concentrate on effective use of time. These behaviors can entail setting goals, planning tasks, prioritizing, and formulating "to-do" lists and group tasks.
3. Monitoring behaviors wherein persons observe their own use of time while involved in activities. This observation is then used to generate a feedback loop that permits a limit on interruptions from other individuals.

Chase and colleagues (2013) talk about a trinity of factors that can derail a person's ability to effectively manage time to develop a research program. This trinity includes procrastination, attending to interruptions, and lack of discipline. Chase et al. (2013) provided the following strategies researchers can use to decline requests that would decrease their scholarship productivity:

- Do not give an immediate decision so you have time to consider whether the request fits into your priorities
- State that you are not the right individual for the request
- Blame your mentor if your mentor supports being blamed
- Express your gratitude for being asked, but respectfully decline
- Do not provide specific excuses for declining the offer
- Explore whether some trade-offs can be made to be able to accept the request

The editorial board members of the *Western Journal of Nursing Research* shared their own time management strategies that helped to contribute to their research success (Chase et al., 2013). Table 5.1 presents their strategies for time management, namely, setting realistic and attainable goals, optimizing realistic planning, prioritizing, effective scheduling, maintaining focus on research program, involving a team, rewarding yourself for achievement, managing potential distractions, problem solving and managing barriers, balancing life, and analyzing progress and time management strategies periodically.

The following is some sage advice from Austin (2001) about developing a research program:

> If you have a realistic idea of the struggles of doing research, then you won't quit when things do not go well for you. I think one of the major reasons we have too few nurse researchers is that they are not prepared for the struggles, they become discouraged, and they quit before they really get started. (p. 173)

- **TABLE 5.1 Time Management Strategies**

Strategy	Implementing Time Management Strategy

Set realistic and attainable goals	• Develop long-term scholarship goals
	• Develop intermediate and immediate activities to achieve long-term goals
	• Link goals with a defined process
	• Identify goals/objectives that are measurable and attainable within a structured time limit
	• Determine what is under your direct control as you will have the most ability to achieve these goals
	• Periodically review goals for
	  ■ Achievement/lack of achievement
	  ■ Factors that facilitate or impede achievement

(continued)

• **TABLE 5.1 Time Management Strategies** *(continued)*

Strategy	Implementing Time Management Strategy
Optimize realistic planning	• Create daily "to-do" lists and check off tasks as they are done • Break complex tasks, such as manuscripts, into manageable components with defined deadlines • Amass resources prior to beginning a task • Create a detailed timeline of activities • When you end your work session, make an agenda of "to-do" items for the next session while it is fresh in your mind • When you finish a writing session, jot down notes of what to write in the next paragraphs • Automate some processes (e.g., sign up to receive automated notices of funding opportunities or research papers) • Identify and seek needed assistance early in the process • Use an electronic file management system for an organized approach to work
Prioritize	• Acknowledge the primacy of your work • Arrange your objectives/goals in order of priority • Work on highest-priority goal first and consistently until you have achieved the goal or have temporarily exhausted available resources • Write down priorities—if request or opportunity is not in line with priority, say "no" • Learn when and how to say "no"
Effective scheduling	• Schedule blocks of writing time • Schedule far in advance of deadlines • Choose days that tend to be less demanding than other days of the week • Create a recurring schedule with scholarship blocks • Use an electronic calendar • Make electronic calendar available to others so they may see your availability (outside times blocked for scholarly productivity) • When meeting with others, schedule time-limited appointments • Consider scheduling a "research sabbatical" aimed at completing selected research tasks
Maintain focus on research program	• Select opportunities that advance research program (e.g., student work, commitments) • Engage your clinical teaching and service in support of your science • Remove undue drifting to other "interesting topics" • Develop a way to work with multiple students on one project that also contributes to your program of research

(continued)

● TABLE 5.1 Time Management Strategies *(continued)*

Strategy	Implementing Time Management Strategy
Involve a team	• Delegate work to divide labor among team members • Seek early peer review for potential revisions • Actively enlist support to facilitate research productivity at the school level
Reward yourself for achievement	• Plan rewards for "to-do's" • Reward completion of parts of large projects instead of waiting until the entire project is finished

Manage potential distractions	• Create a work environment that is free from external distractions
	  ■ Schedule work in a "secure" or cloistered setting
	  ■ Create a physical space where you keep your materials "set up" and ready
	• Turn off visual and auditory interruptions (e.g., e-mail/text alerts, phone)
	• Determine potential internal distractions and create a separate list so when these distractions develop, they can be briefly recorded and dismissed from thought to focus on the work at hand
	• Avoid multitasking as this leads to unnecessary distractions and does not increase productivity

Problem solve and manage barriers	• Honestly appraise barriers • Discuss possible solutions with mentors and peers • Trial barriers management strategies and assess for effectiveness
Balancing life	• Get adequate rest, sleep, and regular physical activity • Set aside time for relaxation and downtime
Analyze progress and time management strategies periodically	• Reassess research productivity after instituting potential solutions—continuous quality improvement • Reassess major goals at least quarterly • Consider using "productivity" or "project management" software

Reprinted with permission from Chase et al. (2013, pp. 157–158).

INTERDISCIPLINARY COLLABORATIVE RESEARCH

Collaborative, interdisciplinary research can be a valuable component of a program of research. In a research trajectory, there is no need to walk down a path alone. Collaboration is "a process by which members of various disciplines share their expertise. Accomplishing this requires that these individuals understand and appreciate what it is that they contribute to the whole" (Henneman, 1995, p. 363). Collaborative research can range from persons working on different components of the research project fairly isolated from each other, to members of a team working on all components of the project together, starting with the conception of the research study to writing up manuscripts of the results. In addition, there are a myriad of configurations possible for a team research project. Collaborative efforts can be between different professional groups, such as academics and health care providers, or between different organizations, or between different disciplines. For any one project at any time, one or all of these different collaborative levels may come into play. Richardson (2006) used the term "de-disciplining" to capture the process of involving researchers from different disciplines to study complex problems. Looking beyond our disciplinary boundaries is at the heart of this type of research. To promote contemporary mixed methods research, Freshwater (2014) calls for incentivized inclusiveness and focused diversity so that multiple truths can coexist and have an opportunity to flourish.

Hall et al. (2006) defined interdisciplinary health research (IDHR) as "a team of researchers, solidly grounded in their respective disciplines, that come together around an important and challenging health issue, the research question for which is determined by a shared understanding in an interactive and iterative process" (p. 764). Hall and colleagues (2006) emphasized that "interdisciplinary scholarship requires the deconstruction of knowledge and identity, which is then reconfigured into new forms of knowledge and action. Researchers working in interdisciplinary realms must demonstrate the ability to move between interdisciplinary and disciplinary scholarship" (p. 764).

Barriers to interdisciplinary health research are distinct disciplinary identities where the distinctive culture of each discipline flourishes. Academic organizational structures help to entrench these distinctive identities via resource allocation, such as budgets and space allocation (Hall et al., 2006). Complicating further the facilitation of interdisciplinary research are agencies outside academia, such as granting agencies.

The need for collaboration in our discipline of nursing is particularly important because of the complexity of issues our patients must contend with. If researchers remain in their own subspecialties, they may not even be aware of these complex issues. McCorkle (2011a) emphasized that a team of interdisciplinary experts should comprise not only methodological and analytical experts but also conceptual and clinical experts. The mere fact that each member of the team is an expert in a particular field does not ensure a successful collaborative team. These experts need to complement each other and appreciate each other's expertise. McCorkle stressed that the interdisciplinary team members may need to view their own disciplines in a new light, with an attitude of humility to reconsider concepts with insights from the other disciplines represented in the team. A benefit of collaboration is that it can result in researchers thinking in innovative ways rather than within the traditional paradigms of their own disciplines. When clinicians are included in the collaborative team, they help to bridge the gap between research and practice.

Lancaster (1985) identified the collaborative research process as including the six Cs: contributions, communication, commitment, consensus, compatibility, and credit. Each individual on the research team should be recruited for the unique contribution that he or she can make by his or her individual expertise. Communication among team members is essential for a successful collaboration. Commitment is both physical and emotional, and the same level of commitment among team members is ideal. Researchers on the team need to appreciate each other's differences and find ways to create harmony. Respect for each other is also necessary to achieve not only compatibility but also consensus. Lancaster warned that credit in a collaborative research project can be problematic. Who gets credit for what? This issue of credit is critical for promotion and tenure. These six Cs comprise a never-ending process during the course of the project.

D'Amour, Ferrada-Videla, Rodriguez, and Beaulieu (2005) defined collaboration according to five underlying concepts: sharing, partnership, power, interdependency, and process. These authors go on to state that the most complete collaborative models are based on a theoretical background. Keleher (1998) described successful collaborative research as incorporating effective communication, active listening, true dialogue, being aware of and appreciating differences, and capability to negotiate options.

Bammer (2008) explored three areas of research collaboration that address three key management challenges. The first is to effectively harness differences, which are of two types. One relates to integrating varied relevant contributions, and the other to preventing issues that arise from attributes that are incidental to the team collaboration. Bammer identified a structural approach of questions for describing how integration is arrived at. Collaborators on a research team need to ask themselves: What will they integrate? In what context will the integration take place? Who will do the integration? What method will be used?

The second key management challenge is to set defensible boundaries in terms of disciplinary and practice perspectives. Bammer (2008) identified a set of questions that are offered as a starting point for the team's discussion. Examples of these questions are as follows:

- What can the collaborators from different academic disciplines contribute to the research study?
- Are there any contentious issues involved in this cross-disciplinary research?
- Are there any political, social, or cultural issues that need to be addressed?

The third area of research collaboration is to gain legitimate authorization. The current diverse sources of research funding and collaboration require additional authorization. This authorization can come at a cost to research independence. In designing a collaborative project, researchers need to work out the type and level of authorization required, and how to obtain it with minimal strings attached.

McCorkle (2011a) identified four key steps to successful collaboration in research:

1. Right from the beginning, routine meetings should be held. All the researchers in the collaborative team should be polled to obtain the best times they can meet. Once the time that fits best with all the researchers' schedules has been decided, the times for the meetings should be made consistent throughout the research project. These regularly scheduled meetings are key to fostering collaboration and to providing opportunities to discuss any issues regarding the study.
2. A different type of meeting may also be necessary if the research involves vulnerable populations and patients who are suffering. This work is emotionally draining and can take a toll on the study's staff involved in providing the intervention being tested or in collecting the data with patients. Periodic team meetings or support groups can help the staff cope with their own distress in caring for patients in the research situations. Support groups will not only help the staff in coping but also ensure retention of the staff throughout the research project. For example, loss of trained data collectors can set the research back as new staff need to be recruited and also trained.
3. If the collaborative research involves an intervention, then fidelity of the intervention is critical and needs continuous monitoring throughout the research. Periodic meetings of the research staff to discuss quality assurance aspects of the intervention can help to ensure adherence to the intervention protocols.
4. The last key to successful collaboration is the infrastructure in the research setting. It is desirable to have a formal research center at the institution with designated administrative staff to support the management of the research project.

The following checklist has been developed by McCorkle (2011a) to ensure successful collaboration:

- Review team of experts, and add collaborators where deficits exist.
- Build long-term collaborations based on trust, humility, and kinship.
- Forge pre- and poststudy networks across disciplines and settings.
- Establish a schedule of separate meetings within each key component of study.
- Form a support group/structure for staff.

- Review grant resources, and request shared resources within your institutions.
- Monitor intervention for consistency and effects.
- Advocate for an institutional infrastructure geared toward collaboration. (McCorkle, 2011a, p. 542)

"Interdisciplinary work spans the complex intellectual and institutional boundaries of the disciplines" (Giacomini, 2004, p. 178). Dreams of interdisciplinary work can, however, turn into nightmares, some of which have been highlighted by Giacomini: One is the specialty language of each discipline. A common language among researchers on a team in different disciplines is needed or else the dream of interdisciplinary work will be turned into team meetings that look like the towers of Babel. Another potential nightmare stems from each discipline creating its own separate island of knowledge and not recognizing the relevant knowledge of the other disciplines on the team. Disciplinary blinders need to be removed so that new collaborations among researchers can yield unique methods of discovery.

Giacomini (2004) also identified some interdisciplinary maladies and potential remedies. The first is what is called "bandwagon sickness," where researchers jump on the interdisciplinary bandwagon before they know where it is going. With the allure of interdisciplinary research funding, researchers may find themselves on research teams where the match is not right for them. Smart choices need to be made. As Giacomini stated, "[S]elective matchmaking should pursue interdisciplinarity rather than any-disciplinarity" (p. 180).

A second interdisciplinary malady is 101 Exasperation. Giacomini (2004) proposed that this occurs from team members' weariness and depressive symptoms as they have to keep establishing common ground with each new collaborator to the team. "Constant stirring can destroy interdisciplinary work that has just begun to gel" (Giacomini, 2004, p. 181). Retreats, workshops, and playfulness were offered as some remedies.

The last malady Giacomini (2004) identified was adisciplinarity, which entails "the experience of leaving well-forged channels and finding one's research programme at sea" (p. 181). It involves questioning just where this new interdisciplinary knowledge lies. What journals are appropriate for the submission of articles for publication? Which conferences to now attend?

Collaborative research has much to offer our discipline of nursing; however, it can be fraught with problematic issues stemming from the political nature of collaboration (Beattie, Cheek, & Gibson, 1996). The politics of collaboration operates on multiple levels, such as the individual level and the institutional level. Beattie and colleagues alerted nurse researchers to the "invisible political dimension" (p. 683) in collaboration where power relations occur within the team. Beattie et al. (1996) used Brookfield's (1993) themes of impostorship, cultural suicide, and road running as the theoretical framework for their discussion of the politics of collaborative research. Impostorship is experienced by some nurses when they feel they are not qualified for the task at hand, in this case, collaborative research. They feel they are presenting a false self and asking themselves what they have to offer this research project. If collaborative research is to be successful, team members need to be supported to share their real or perceived limitations. Unequal distribution of power can result if the collaborative nature of the project is not supported by all team members.

Cultural suicide is another of Brookfield's (1993) themes, which involves reactions of others to nurses collaborating in an interdisciplinary research project. Here, the nurses risk being cut off from their disciplinary or organizational culture. Collaboration needs to be viewed as not defecting to another side but instead as working with others to better achieve a goal. Feelings of being marginalized from peers can take a toll on team members.

Lastly, road running is a metaphor that describes the ups and downs that team members experience during the collaborative research process. Beattie et al. (1996) shared that during their large-scale funded collaborative nursing research study, at times the members were overwhelmed with the sense of taking one step forward and then three steps back. Beattie and colleagues stressed that to ignore the political dimensions of collaborative research can potentially jeopardize the entire research project.

EXEMPLARS OF NURSE RESEARCHERS' COLLABORATIVE RESEARCH TEAMS

Nurse researchers have been successful in traversing this rocky path of collaborative research. To illustrate, first, I will share my own experience with an interdisciplinary team of researchers. Next, two examples are provided to illustrate intradisciplinary research teams, plus one example of interdisciplinary research teams of other nurse researchers.

In my program of research, an interdisciplinary collaborative research team was necessary to conduct my double-blind, randomized control trial to study the effect of maternal DHA supplementation during pregnancy on reducing symptoms of postpartum depression. Together with Dr. Carol Lammi Keefe, a PhD in nutritional sciences, we secured a grant from a private foundation, the Patrick and Katherine Weldon Donaghue Medical Research Foundation, to conduct this study. In addition to the two of us, the team consisted of a postdoc in nutritional sciences, another PhD in nutrition, and a PhD student in nursing. As can be seen in Figure 5.2, this study entailed a complex, longitudinal design of data collection and analysis. In addition, we also had a number of staff persons to help with data collection, such as a phlebotomist, to go into the mothers' homes to draw blood samples, and staff nurses at the hospital and private obstetricians' offices to help recruit mothers for the

• **FIGURE 5.2 DHA Timeline**

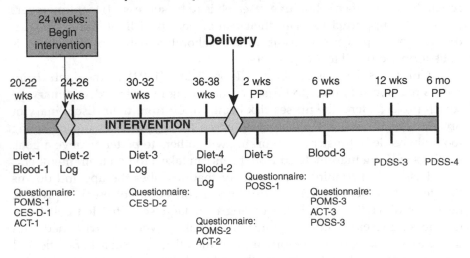

Postpartum Depression Prevention Project

study. All the members on my interdisciplinary team were a dream to work with. Thank goodness, however, I had budgeted funds from the grant to hire a grants manager, because the amount of time and effort to coordinate this study, the recruitment and data collection, was immense.

Pamela Hinds

In the beginning of Hinds' research program on fatigue in children and adolescents diagnosed with cancer, she collaborated with staff nurses who provided direct patient care at two children's cancer centers, one in Texas and the other in Tennessee (Hinds, Ruccione, & Kelly, 1997). Hinds purposely collaborated with these nurses not only to help with data collection but also to foster their enthusiasm for clinical research. Hinds called these nurses fatigue clinical nurse scholars. The aim of the initial study in Hinds' research program was to develop conceptual definitions of fatigue in this population (Hinds & Hockenberry-Eaton, 2001). A series of focus groups were held with patients, parents, and staff members to obtain each group's perspectives on fatigue in the pediatric oncology patient. Each fatigue clinical nurse scholar attended a half-day workshop on focus group interviews. At the workshop, the nurses practiced the roles of focus group moderator and observer. In addition to running focus groups, the fatigue clinical nurse scholars developed and field-tested two age-specific educational tools for children and adolescent cancer patients' fatigue.

Judith Wuest and Colleagues

A collaborative team approach to building knowledge about women's health and violence was used: Marilyn Ford-Gilboe, Marilyn Merritt-Gray, Colleen Varcoe, and Judith Wuest, all nurse researchers, have collaborated for more than a decade to explore women's health in the context of intimate partner violence (IPV) in three Canadian provinces, British Columbia (BC), Ontario (ON), and New Brunswick (NB). The unique expertise of each member has allowed this team to logically respond to research questions as they emerge from each successive project using appropriate research approaches such as qualitative theory development, quantitative survey research, intervention development, and intervention feasibility and efficacy testing.

Their initial grounded theory research generated two theories. The first, *Reclaiming Self*, captured women's proactive process of leaving abusive partners (Merritt-Gray & Wuest, 1995; Wuest & Merritt-Gray, 1999). The second, *Strengthening Capacity to Limit Intrusion (SCLI)*, portrays how women and their children promote their health after leaving an abusive household through the processes of rebuilding security and providing, renewing, and regenerating family that help limit intrusion (Ford-Gilboe, Wuest, & Merritt-Gray, 2005). Intrusion, the basic social problem for families trying to promote their health, was defined as pervasive interference from ongoing abuse, physical and mental health problems, "costs" of seeking help, and negative lifestyle changes (Wuest, Ford-Gilboe, Merritt-Gray, & Berman, 2003). The *SCLI* highlighted the fallacy that leaving an abusive partner solves the problems of IPV for women, as well as the gap in services for women beyond the crisis of leaving. Further, the range of participant health problems that were found to interfere with women's ability to promote their health illuminated the paucity of knowledge regarding the trajectory of women's health after leaving. Consequently, the researchers embarked on the women's health effects study (WHES) with a community sample of 309 women who had separated from abusive partners within the previous 3 years. The WHES was a longitudinal 4-year quantitative study documenting annual changes in women's health; abuse experiences; personal, social, and economic resources; and service use (Ford-Gilboe et al., 2009). Data provided a rich resource for understanding patterns, mediators, and consequences of diverse aspects of women's health and resources after leaving. For example, using structural equation modeling, Wuest et al. (2010) found that the severity of assaultive and psychological IPV and child abuse mediated by lifetime abuse-related injury, PTSD symptom severity, and depressive symptom severity accounted for 40.2% of the variance in women's chronic pain severity. Varcoe et al. (2011), in a costing analysis of resources used by women, found the total annual costs of public and private health and social services attributable to violence to be $13,162 per woman. These analyses, the *SCLI* theory and the paucity of health services available for women after leaving, were catalysts for the development of the Intervention for Health Enhancement After Leaving (*iHeal;* Figure 5.3 and Table 5.2; Ford-Gilboe, Merritt-Gray, Varcoe, & Wuest, 2011).

Both qualitative and quantitative data are useful for modifying a grounded theory (Glaser & Strauss, 1967). The team used the quantitative data from the WHES and extant theoretical and practice literature as secondary data for theoretical sampling as they modified the original *SCLI* theory and used constant comparative analysis to move from explanatory theory to a theoretical construction of how best to practice in the *iHEAL* (Wuest, Ford-Gilboe, Merritt-Gray, & Varcoe, 2013). The *iHEAL* is a 6-month primary health care intervention designed to be provided by a nurse and a domestic violence (DV) support worker. The goal of the *iHEAL* is to improve the quality of life, health, and capacity of women who have left abusive partners while reducing their intrusion. Feasibility studies for the *iHEAL* have been completed recently in NB and ON. The NB study took place in two rural and two urban communities with nurses hired to partner with the existing DV outreach workers in providing the *iHEAL*. In ON, the setting was a metropolitan area, and implementation was primarily by nurses with support from a social worker. Feasibility and preliminary efficacy findings from both studies are promising. In BC, the *iHEAL* is being adapted for implementation with women in an indigenous context, and efficacy testing is beginning with a sample of urban Aboriginal women.

Importantly, collaborators on this team not only draw on each member's philosophical and methodological expertise but also act as mentors to one another. Merritt-Gray's experience as a community mental health nurse working with women in abusive relationships was a catalyst for the initial study, and her strong practice lens keeps the team mindful of clinical

• **FIGURE 5.3 Theory of Strengthening Capacity to Limit Intrusion**

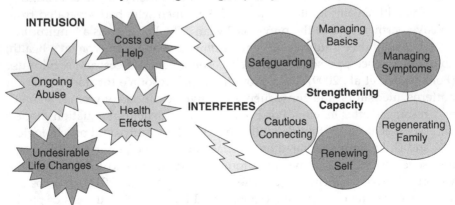

Reprinted with permission from Ford-Gilboe et al. (2011, p. 203).

significance and meaning. In the grounded theory research, Wuest supported Merritt-Gray and Ford-Gilboe in learning to "do" grounded theory. In the WHES study, Ford-Gilboe supported Wuest's efforts to make the shift to quantitative research design, particularly by critiquing her quantitative manuscripts. Varcoe's critical lens frames IPV within broader social, political, and historical relations, and supports the team in increasing awareness of and challenging dominant Eurocentric assumptions and values. The collective growth from their diverse expertise positions the team well to take on new challenges such as the development and testing of the *iHEAL*.

Ruth McCorkle

McCorkle (2011b) is a strong proponent of interdisciplinary collaboration. As she stated, "It is only by working with others to study common

• **TABLE 5.2** "Intervention for Health Enhancement After Leaving" (iHEAL) Components

Safeguarding	Assisting the woman with limiting her exposure and that of her family to people or circumstances that threaten their physical and emotional safety, by assessing her sense of safety and developing strategies to manage risks and build her sense of security.
Managing basics	Assisting the woman with securing and building economic, material, and personal energy resources needed to establish and sustain herself separate from the abuser over time.
Managing symptoms	Supporting the woman to identify her most intrusive symptoms and health problems and to build confidence in preventing and managing symptoms, through both self-care strategies and support from health professionals.
Cautious connecting	Supporting the woman to enhance her instrumental support, sense of belonging, and social connection by evaluating the costs and optimizing the benefits of current and potential relationships with peers, extended family, social networks, or formal service agencies.
Renewing self	Helping the woman turn inward and focus on personal restoration, making meaning of her past, and working toward a more personally fulfilling future.
Regenerating family	Family "storyline," finding functional ways to work together to meet everyday needs in a predictable way through rules, routines, and new roles, and purposefully developing new constructive ways of getting along as a family unit or team.

Reprinted with permission from Ford-Gilboe et al. (2011, p. 208).

problems from varied perspectives that our research grows. By broadening one's own perspective, it logically follows that interdisciplinary activities increase including publishing in non-nursing journals and participating in multidisciplinary organizations through poster and paper presentations" (pp. 337–338). Table 5.3 provides some examples of McCorkle's collaborations with other investigators during her program of research.

• **TABLE 5.3 Examples of McCorkle's Contributions to Science Through Collaboration**

Author/Year	Study	Citation
Mock et al. (1998)	Establishing mechanisms to conduct multi-institutional research-fatigue in patients with cancer: An exercise intervention	*Oncology Nursing Forum, 5*(8), 1391–1397
Norman et al. (2001)	Development and validation of a telephone questionnaire to measure lymphedema in women treated for breast cancer	*Physical Therapy, 81*(6), 1192–1205
Given et al. (2002)	Pain and fatigue management: Results of a nursing randomized clinical trial	*Oncology Nursing Forum, 29*(6), 949–956
Given et al. (2004)	Effect of a cognitive behavioral intervention on reducing symptom severity during chemotherapy	*Journal of Clinical Oncology, 22*(3), 507–516
Mock et al. (2005)	Exercise manages fatigue during breast cancer treatment: A randomized controlled trial	*Psycho-Oncology, 14*, 464–477
Sikorskii et al. (2006)	Testing the effects of treatment complications on a cognitive behavioral intervention for reducing symptom severity	*Journal of Pain Symptom Management, 32*(2), 129–139
Greenwald et al. (2008)	Health status and adaptation among long-term cervical cancer survivors	*Gynecologic Oncology, 111*(3), 449–454
Wolpin et al. (2008)	Acceptability of an electronic self-report assessment program for patients with cancer	*Computers, Informatics, Nursing, 26*(6), 332–338

(continued)

• TABLE 5.3 Examples of McCorkle's Contributions to Science Through Collaboration (*continued*)

Author/Year	Study	Citation
Greenwald and McCorkle (2008)	Sexuality and sexual functions in long-term survival of cervical cancer	*Journal of Women's Health, 17*(6), 955–963
Fann et al. (2009)	Depression screening using the Patient Health Questionnaire 9 administered on a touch screen computer	*Psycho-Oncology, 18*(1), 14–22
Ferrucci et al. (2011)	Causal attribution among cancer survivors of the 10 most common cancers	*Journal of Psycho-social Oncology, 29*(2), 121–140
Berry et al. (2011)	Enhancing patient-provider communication with the electronic self-report assessment for cancer: A randomized trial	*Journal of Clinical Oncology, 29*(8), 1029–1035
Kim et al. (2011)	Quality of life among testicular cancer survivors: A case-control study in the United States	*Quality of Life Research, 20*(10), 1629–1637
Yu et al. (2012)	Employment experiences of cancer survivors of 2 years post-diagnosis in the study of cancer survivors	*Journal of Cancer Survivorship, 6*(2), 210–218
Fletcher et al. (2013)	Gender differences in the evaluation of illness understanding among patients with advanced cancer	*Journal of Supportive Oncology, 11*(3), 126–132
Wagner et al. (2013)	Nurse navigators in early cancer care: A randomized controlled trial	*Journal of Clinical Oncology, 32*(11), 12–18

QUALITATIVE INTERDISCIPLINARY COLLABORATION

Strategies to guide qualitative teamwork based on mutual adjustment are offered by Hall et al. (2006). Reflexivity is a key strategy. Important is the team members specifying their presumptions and biases regarding the research. Hall and colleagues used two reflexive exercises. In the first exercise, members of the qualitative team wrote out their preferences and biases based on their life experiences. Team members also shared their stakes in the research project, their theoretical lens, and the findings they expect from this qualitative study. The aim of this exercise was to identify how team members' differences may affect the data collection and analysis processes.

The second exercise emphasized key theoretical concepts that team members believed might be related to categories that would be identified from data analysis. Hall et al. (2006) shared how the team's enhanced theoretical sensitivity helped to acknowledge their varied perspectives and to evaluate the usefulness of their concepts. The reflexivity exercises provided a solid basis for the iterative process of data analysis in Hall and colleagues' qualitative research.

In a later study, Hall (2011) recruited an interdisciplinary team to conduct a constructivist, feminist narrative study to describe the trauma recovery process in 44 women who survived childhood maltreatment. Members of this interdisciplinary team represented nursing, psychology, psychiatry, and women's studies. The purposes of this qualitative study were to describe the "(a) aftereffects of trauma, (b) strengths and strategies used in recovery, (c) helpful key relationships and related social interactions, and (d) the social, cultural, and political contexts of the participants' narratives" (p. 4). This interdisciplinary team constructed a trauma recovery process they entitled "becoming resolute," which incorporated key relationships, life trajectories, self-strategies, and perceptual changes.

Barry, Britten, Barber, Bardley, and Stevenson (1999) proposed that reflexivity be thought of not just as an individual activity but also as a team activity. The team sharing of reflexive writing and its resulting group discussion can facilitate a research team's productivity, its functioning in qualitative research, and its rigor. Qualitative teamwork can facilitate a higher level of conceptual thinking than researchers working individually can. Team members from different disciplines can provide a wider base from which to view qualitative data than one individual representing one discipline. Another benefit of qualitative teamwork is the emotional support members can provide each other.

Barry and colleagues (1999), however, identified some pitfalls of qualitative teamwork of which researchers need to be cognizant. One such pitfall is the cult of individualism in academia. Promotion and tenure focus on individual achievement, first authorship, and so forth, which can hinder successful qualitative teamwork. Problems can surface at both ends of the continuum, with either too much agreement, where individuals are unwilling to share their true feelings, or too much competition, where team meetings are filled with endless disagreement over trivial matters.

Qualitative research, being fluid and emergent, can lead to some team members becoming uncomfortable and insecure. Personal negotiation skills and conflict resolution are helpful for individual team members to work together. Achieving group consensus in all phases of a qualitative project is a time-consuming process. Providing opportunities for all team members to share their ideas can be frustrating and painful. Collaborative writing can also be problematic.

When evaluating the effectiveness of a qualitative research team, we need to look at not only project outcomes but also the team members' satisfaction and function. According to West (1994), a high level of reflexivity is required to achieve a fully functioning team.

Barry and colleagues (1999) shared the reflexive tools they used to help raise awareness of the orientation of the team members and also to aid the process of communicating and negotiating to arrive at group consensus such as group discussions, reflexive writing, awareness of differences, and negotiation. One of their reflexive tools involved each team member writing and sharing answers to orientation questions such as the following:

- In what way might my experience color my participation in the project?
- What experience have I had with qualitative research?
- What theoretical lens do I favor to apply to the results? (p. 35)

Barry had done this exercise at the first team meeting, but suggested that this may have been too early. The team had not had time to bond yet or to trust each other, and the exercise caused some anxiety.

With more hierarchical qualitative research teams emerging, Rogers-Dillon (2005) addressed issues pertinent to the power dynamics and ethical uses involved when qualitative knowledge is produced in these social contexts. Rogers-Dillon's interest in this topic stems from her hierarchical qualitative research teams that involved a graduate research assistant. Tensions that can occur in hierarchical qualitative research teams can consume valuable research time. Rogers-Dillon offered the following suggestions for minimizing the impact these tensions can have on the qualitative research team:

- Make power dynamics explicit.
- Have an ethics clause. Research assistants should not violate their personal ethics to follow the study protocol.
- Separate out collaboration where the data collection and collaboration are separate and sequential.
- Clarify what is social.
- Institute hazard pay where qualitative researchers often endure hardships and hazard.
- Pay for breaks where research assistants get paid for 1 to 2 hours per week for off time to help release any pressure that may develop during fieldwork.
- Institute theoretical memos that allow research assistants to process what they have been observing.

Lingard, Schryer, Spafford, and Campbell (2007) explored the politics of identity in a qualitative interdisciplinary health research team. Over their 5 years of working together, they addressed lessons learned that they hope will assist other interdisciplinary teams to reach their full potential. Unlike Rogers-Dillon (2005), who addressed hierarchical qualitative research teams, Lingard and colleagues focused on collaborations among established researchers. Following Barry et al.'s (1999) assertion of the necessity of both individual and team reflexivity, Lingard and colleagues used three sociological theories on which to base their reflexive exercise: (a) Wenger's (1998) concept of knowledge brokers, (b) Bourdieu and Wacquant's (1992) cultural and symbolic capital notion, and (c) Giddens's (1993) theory of structuration. The concept of knowledge broker addresses the individual experiences of researchers in inhabiting and crossing disciplinary boundaries. Cultural and symbolic capital refers to various forms of capital that must be negotiated as members of the team work together. Giddens's structuration informs researchers on how structures in our organizations and ideologies support but also constrain our collaborative research.

Lingard et al. (2007) suggest three lessons their research team learned. The first is the need to explicitly negotiate the tensions that may exist in member identities. If these tensions are not worked through in the qualitative research team, they can undermine the coherence of the team. The second is to clearly articulate the research team's logic of practice to new members of the team instead of expecting newcomers to intuit it by means of the work process. The third lesson focuses on writing as an interdisciplinary qualitative team and just how complex shaping knowledge in a manuscript is. Team members need to be cognizant of how the politics of identity on the team shapes the politics of writing up qualitative findings.

With the push of funding agencies toward interdisciplinary research and also mixed methods research, Morse (2008) warned that "the trend toward team and collaborative research is of dubious good for qualitative inquiry" (p. 4). She expressed concern that these larger collaborative teams may dilute qualitative inquiry and make compromises that will not benefit qualitative research. Morse asserts that "we must retain control of our data and control of our analysis and not be smothered by quantitative styles. We must retain our value of theoretical development over speed" (p. 4).

In order to do excellent qualitative research, there are two qualitative data collection and analysis difficulties that need to be addressed in collaborative research. The first is what Morse called the "making" of excellent qualitative data. Excellent interview data depend on the skill of the interviewer. Second, how does the principal investigator "get inside the head" of the research assistants who have collected the data? In collaborative qualitative research, there is the danger of diluting the qualitative data and of making compromises that might not be in the best interests of qualitative research.

Morse (2008) identified six styles of collaboration for large group qualitative projects, each of which has its advantages and disadvantages.

1. "Cohesive" involves most of the team recording and analyzing the interviews. This style of collaboration can provide rich insights into the findings, but it can lengthen the research process if busy team members have difficulty making scheduled meetings.
2. "Split the domain" involves dividing the parts of the project into smaller pieces.
3. "Providing summaries" involves the team member who has done the interviews reporting to the group a summary of the participants' experiences.
4. In "skill level assignment," the principal investigator assigns the research team different tasks such as interviewing or coding the data. Morse warns that this is a dangerous style to use. If the principal investigator entrusts the interviewing or coding to a research assistant, who may not be skilled enough, the entire research study can be jeopardized.
5. "Convenience style" depends on the amount of time the principal investigator has to devote to the study. The principal investigator may assign some of the tasks at times to a research assistant. The quality of the research may be affected.
6. The last style of collaboration was not named by Morse because she was uncertain what to label it. With this style most of the project is done by research assistants. Morse warns that if the research is interpretive in nature, the project may be a waste of time.

Problems in pacing and communication may occur since the efficiency of group work in qualitative inquiry does not approach that in quantitative research (Morse, 2008). The quantitative researchers on a team may not be familiar with the slower pace of good qualitative inquiry. Larger teams may not have the same degree of commitment from all their members, leading to power struggles. Interpretive qualitative research, more than quantitative research, further complicates matters where analysis of data is not so straightforward.

Cheek (2008) asked, "Is collaboration a desirable and useful goal for the qualitative researchers?" (p. 1600). We cannot take for granted that collaboration has all positive aspects. Qualitative researchers need to pause, reflect, and consider what assumptions underpin whatever is discussed in the collaboration. We should not just focus on whom to collaborate with and what we will collaborate about. The politics of research collaboration cannot be dismissed. Cheek purports that "collaboration viewed in this way is thus a matter of strategy and of strategic positioning, both of qualitative research itself and of qualitative researchers" (p. 1601). In collaborative research, the qualitative portion should not routinely be seen as the precursor to the quantitative project or just a small piece that is used to enhance the quantitative results.

Cheek (2008) asked qualitative researchers, "How can, in our research collaboration, we remain faithful to the [tenets] of qualitative inquiry yet be mindful of connections and disconnections, contradictions and paradoxes, within the contemporary context in which we conduct that research?" (p. 1602). She goes on to say, "How to navigate this potentially fraught pathway replete with tensions between the expedient and the ideal, the non-negotiable and the negotiable, to find a place where we can feel comfortable as qualitative researchers is one of the key implications and challenges arising for qualitative researchers" when collaborating (p. 1602).

INTERNATIONAL RESEARCH COLLABORATION

International research collaboration in nursing is critical for addressing global health care issues and reducing disparities among vulnerable populations. It is, however, a complex and fragile process. First, the benefits of international research collaboration are described followed by the challenges.

Rolfe et al. (2004) stressed that the power of international collaboration in research lies in the opportunity to compare experiences, methods, and data analysis. Freshwater, Sherwood, and Drury (2006) described the benefits of sharing methods and protocols in their international research collaboration. Their assumptions were challenged and led to new perspectives and learning different research skills that had been unique to one region. The power of international collaboration also lies in advancing the global health care agenda. It can transform health care as researchers are able to test interventions with multiple populations at the same time (Freshwater et al., 2006).

Freshwater and colleagues (2006) outlined the barriers and challenges to successful international partnerships in research, such as financial costs, language, differences, intellectual property rights, and differing time zones. Examples of financial costs can include travel, telephone and videoconferencing, and hiring of translators. Budget management can present challenges as these practices can vary from country to country. Rules may be different regarding how monies can be used. Travel costs may be reduced by means of telephone and videoconferencing, but researchers need to negotiate how these costs will be shared across the universities. Language differences can add another set of barriers. For instance, words with different meanings in different countries can lead to misunderstandings not only among the researchers but also with the research participants. Grant writing can also be challenging if the research team has different languages as their primary language. Training data collectors in another country through videoconferencing presents challenges. The success of research relies on fidelity to the intervention.

Freshwater et al. (2006) addressed the potential problems with subject recruitment, which can vary from country to country. Different cultural beliefs and practices can impact the way subjects may react to our traditional recruitment practices. Grant management can also vary from institution to institution and from country to country, and can present barriers to contract negotiations. Procedures for human subjects review can differ as well as research methods.

Lastly, Freshwater and colleagues (2006) addressed the challenges of various intellectual property rights in different countries. Attitudes can differ regarding plagiarism and ownership. Clear communication about authorship of manuscripts, conference presentations, and so on, is necessary from the start of collaboration.

Acknowledging all these barriers and challenges, Bagshaw, Lepp, and Zorn (2007) stressed that the road to successful international research collaboration can be fraught with bumps, unexpected detours, and, at times, dead ends. Table 5.4 presents roadblocks and counterstrategies for collaboration in research teams, developed by Bagshaw et al. (2007). They offered four key characteristics of successful international research collaboration. The first is acknowledging diversity and developing cooperative goals. Misunderstandings and conflicts can easily develop with research team members coming from different cultural, ethnic, and racial backgrounds. Opportunities to

● **TABLE 5.4 Roadblocks and Counterstrategies for Collaboration in International Research Teams**

Roadblocks to Effective International Teamwork	Strategies to Counteract the Roadblocks and Enhance Effective International Teamwork for Research
Ambivalence and uncertainty	● Develop an inspiring or motivating shared vision ● Establish clear goals and objectives ● Develop clear norms ● Provide access to information and a shared knowledge base to enhance common understanding
Individuals promoting self-interests by working competitively or independently	● Acknowledge diversity, and develop cooperative, shared goals ● Take time and develop trust ● Practice collaborative dialogue ● Empower and recognize all team members' abilities, resources, and strengths ● Focus on the individual and team benefits of mutual, cooperative work ● Share ownership of and responsibility for decisions ● Appreciate all accomplishments

(continued)

• **TABLE 5.4 Roadblocks and Counterstrategies for Collaboration in International Research Teams** (*continued*)

Roadblocks to Effective International Teamwork	Strategies to Counteract the Roadblocks and Enhance Effective International Teamwork for Research
Dynamics that reinforce biases and simplifications, e.g., "groupthink," domination of individual views, demands for conformity, or coalitions formed to promote special interests	• Practice self-reflection and reflectivity • Expose and challenge stereotypes, and respect cultural differences and diversity • Directly and openly confront relationship issues and conflicts as they arise • Engage in constructive, open-minded controversy; explore opposite views, positions, and issues; identify common ground; and generate options and alternatives • Be open to new information and ideas, and be willing to integrate or incorporate different perspectives, ideas, positions, or minority views into effective solutions • Continuously search for opportunities for innovation and be willing to take risks • Be flexible and adaptable when situations change • Communicate for continuous improvement and development

Reprinted with permission from Bagshaw et al. (2007, p. 436).

discuss opposing viewpoints with open minds help team members to recognize and value each other's backgrounds, expertise, and contributions. Discussion also needs to center on developing cooperative goals so that individual and team objectives can be achieved.

The second strategy involves engaging in self-reflection and reflexivity (Bagshaw et al., 2007). In addition to the international research teams critically challenging their values, behaviors, and communication patterns, team members need to be receptive to constructive feedback from other researchers on the team. Bagshaw and colleagues identified the need for self-reflexivity to improve this process. These authors believe that self-reflexivity is not given the time and attention it deserves in facilitating international research collaboration. Each member of the research team should critically examine their own personal and political beliefs and how these can influence their relationships with team members. These influences can range from the person's age, gender, culture, and class, to their spirituality.

Promoting collaborative dialogue is the third strategy offered by Bagshaw et al. (2007). They stressed that one's cultural identity can influence how one approaches dialogue. In meeting the needs and goals of the research team, members representing different countries need to be flexible in adapting to the international dialogue, where language difficulties can arise. Bagshaw and colleagues' fourth strategy for facilitating successful international research collaboration is to take time to develop trust.

Bender et al. (2011) addressed the philosophical/theoretical underpinnings of international research collaboration between low- and high-income countries. Piaget's (1965) concept of social relations of cooperation and constraint was applied to examine international collaboration. The example used was Bender and colleagues' Ethiopian and Canadian research on intimate partner violence in Ethiopia. The most successful international research collaborations are those first understood as social relations between team members who respect and trust each other and can freely discuss researchers' disciplinary and cultural perspectives and power. Bender et al. purport that the perspective of social relations of cooperation provides a shift in research from an exclusive focus on outcomes to reflexive and value-driven collaboration. Bender and colleagues emphasized that the complexities of international research collaboration are magnified when the research involves underresourced and resource-rich countries.

The following is an example from my own program of research with international collaboration. The Perinatal Research and Screening Unit Study in Italy involved my collaboration between the Department of Psychiatry and the Department of Obstetrics and Gynecology at the University of Pisa (Oppo et al., 2009). The aims of this longitudinal study were to identify the frequency of risk factors for postpartum depression listed in the Postpartum Depression Predictors Inventory-Revised (PDPI-Revised) during pregnancy and 1 month postpartum, and to determine the predictive validity of the PDPI-Revised that I had developed earlier in my program of research. Researchers from the Departments of Psychiatry, Neurobiology, Pharmacology, and Biotechnology in the School of Medicine at the University of Pisa; Department of Psychiatry at the School of Medicine at the University of Pittsburgh; and I, at the School of Nursing at the University of Connecticut, comprised this international research team. Women in the study completed my PDPI-Revised at the third and eighth months of pregnancy and again at the first month postpartum. Women were also interviewed postpartum using the Structured Clinical Interview for *DSM-IV* Disorders to determine the presence of major or minor depression. Cutoff scores were identified for this Italian sample. At 1 month after childbirth, the PDPI-Revised predicted 83.4% of postpartum depression.

On the qualitative side of my research trajectory, I collaborated internationally with a nurse researcher in Australia, Dr. Jennieffer Barr. Our phenomenological study explored thoughts of infanticide that did not lead to the act among mothers suffering with postpartum depression (Barr & Beck, 2008).

REFERENCES

Austin, J. K. (2001). Developing a research program. *Journal of the American Psychiatric Nurses Association, 7*(5), 173E–176E.

Bagshaw, D., Lepp, M., & Zorn, C. R. (2007). International research collaboration: Building teams and managing conflicts. *Conflict Resolution Quarterly, 24,* 433–446.

Bammer, G. (2008). Enhancing research collaborations: Three key management challenges. *Research Policy, 37,* 875–887.

Barr, J. A., & Beck, C. T. (2008). Infanticide secrets: Qualitative study on postpartum depression. *Canadian Family Physician, 54,* 1716–1717, e1–e5.

Barry, C. A., Britten, N., Barber, N., Bradley, C., & Stevenson, F. (1999). Using reflexivity to optimize teamwork in qualitative research. *Qualitative Health Research, 9,* 26–44.

Beattie, J., Cheek, J., & Gibson, T. (1996). The politics of collaboration as viewed through the lens of a collaborative nursing research project. *Journal of Advanced Nursing, 24,* 682–687.

Bender, A., Guruge, S., Aga, F., Hailemariam, D., Hyman, I., & Tamiru, M. (2011). International research collaboration as social relation: An Ethiopian-Canadian example. *Canadian Journal of Nursing Research, 43,* 62–75.

Brookfield, S. (1993). On impostorship, cultural suicide, and other dangers: How nurses learn critical thinking. *Journal of Continuing Education in Nursing, 24*(5), 197–205.

Bourdieu, P., & Wacquant, L. (1992). *An invitation to reflexive sociology.* Chicago, IL: University of Chicago Press.

Cheek, J. (2008). Researching collaboratively: Implications for qualitative research and researchers. *Qualitative Health Research, 18*(11), 1599–1603.

Chase, J. A., Topp, R., Smith, C. E., Cohen, M. Z., Fahrenwald, N., Zerwic, J. J., . . . Conn, V. S. (2013). Time management strategies for research productivity. *Western Journal of Nursing Research, 35*(2), 155–176.

Claessens, B. J. C., van Eerde, W., Rutte, C. G., & Roe, R. A. (2007). A review of the time management literature. *Personnel Review, 36*(2), 255–276.

Conn, V. S. (2004). Building a research trajectory. *Western Journal of Nursing Research, 26*(6), 592–594.

D'Amour, D., Ferrada-Videla, M. San Martin Rodriguez, L., & Beaulieu, M. D. (2005). The conceptual basis for interprofessional collaboration: Care concepts and theoretical frameworks. *Journal of Interprofessional Care, 19,* 116–131.

Ford-Gilboe, M., Merritt-Gray, M., Varcoe, C., & Wuest, J. (2011). A theory-based primary health care intervention for women who have left abusive partners. *Advances in Nursing Science, 34,* 198–214.

Ford-Gilboe, M., Wuest, J., & Merritt-Gray, M. (2005). Strengthening capacity to limit intrusion: Theorizing family health promotion in the aftermath of woman abuse. *Qualitative Health Research, 15,* 477–501.

Ford-Gilboe, M., Wuest, J., Varcoe, C., Davies, L., Merritt-Gray, M., Hammerton, J., Wilk, P., & Campbell, J. (2009). Modeling the effects of intimate partner violence and access to resources on women's health in the early years after leaving an abusive partner. *Social Science and Medicine, 68,* 1021–1029.

Freshwater, D. (2014). What counts in mixed methods research: Algorithmic thinking or inclusive leadership? *Journal of Mixed Methods Research, 8*, 327–329.

Freshwater, D., Sherwood, G., & Drury, V. (2006). International research collaboration: Issues, benefits, and challenges of the global network. *Journal of Research in Nursing, 11*, 295–303.

Giacomini, M. (2004). Interdisciplinarity in health services research: Dreams and nightmares, maladies and remedies. *Journal of Health Services Research and Policy, 9*(3), 177–183.

Giddens, A. (1993). Problems of action and structure. In P. Casscell (Ed.), *The Giddens reader* (pp. 88–175). Stanford, CA: Stanford University Press.

Gitlin, L. N., & Lyons, K. J. (2008). *Successful grant writing: Strategies for health and human service professionals.* New York, NY: Springer Publishing Company.

Glaser, B., & Strauss, A. (1967). *The discovery of grounded theory.* Chicago, IL: Aldine.

Hall, J. G., Bainbridge, L., Buchan, A., Cribb, A., Drummond, J., Gyles, T., . . . Solomon, P. (2006). A meeting of minds: Interdisciplinary research in the health sciences in Canada. *Canadian Medical Association Journal, 175*(7), 763–771.

Hall, J. M. (2011). Narrative methods in a study of trauma recovery. *Qualitative Health Research, 21*(1), 3–13.

Henneman, E. A. (1995). Nurse-physician collaboration: A poststructuralist view. *Journal of Advanced Nursing, 22*(2), 359–363.

Hinds, P. S., Ruccione, K., & Kelly, K. P. (1997). Developing intergroup nursing research in pediatric oncology. *Journal of Pediatric Oncology Nursing, 14*(3), 135–136.

Hinds, P. S., & Hockenberry-Eaton, M. (2001). Developing a research program on fatigue in children and adolescents diagnosed with cancer. *Journal of Pediatric Oncology Nursing, 18*(2), 3–12.

Holzemer, W. L. (2009). Building a program of research. *Japan Journal of Nursing Science, 6*, 1–5.

Keleher, K. C. (1998). Collaborative practice: Characteristics, barriers, benefits, and implication for midwifery. *Journal of Nurse Midwifery, 43*(1), 8–11.

Lancaster, J. (1985). The perils and joys of collaborative research. *Nursing Outlook, 33*, 231–232, 238.

Lingard, L., Schryer, C. F., Spafford, M. M., & Campbell, S. L. (2007). Negotiating the politics of identify in an interdisciplinary research team. *Qualitative Research, 7*(4), 501–519.

McCorkle, R. (2011a). Interdisciplinary collaboration in the pursuit of science to improve psychosocial cancer care. *Psycho-Oncology, 20*, 538–543.

McCorkle, R. (2011b). A purposeful career path to make a difference in cancer care. *Cancer Nursing, 34*(4), 335–339.

Merritt-Gray, M., &Wuest, J. (1995). Countering abuse and breaking free: The process of leaving revealed through women's voices. *Health Care for Women International, 16*(5), 399–412.

Morse, J. (2008). Styles of collaboration in qualitative inquiry. *Qualitative Health Research, 18*, 3–4.

Oppo, A., Mauri, M., Ramacciotti, D., Camilleri, V., Banti, C., Borri, C., . . . Cassano, G. B. (2009). Risk factors for postpartum depression: The role of the Postpartum Depression Predictors Inventory-Revised (PDPI-Revised). *Archives of Women's Mental Health, 12*, 239–249.

Piaget, J. (1965). *The moral judgment of the child*. New York, NY: Free Press.

Richardson, L. (2006). Skirting a pleated text: De-disciplining an academic life. In S. Hesse-Biber & P. Leavy (Eds.), *Emergent methods in social research* (pp. 1012). Thousand Oaks, CA: SAGE.

Rogers-Dillon, R. H. (2005). Hierarchical qualitative research teams: Refining the methodology. *Qualitative Research, 5*(4), 437–454.

Rolfe, M. K., Bryar, R. M., Hjelm, K., Apelquist, J., Fletcher, M., & Anderson, B. L. (2004). International collaboration to address common problems in healthcare: Processes, practicalities, and power. *International Nursing Review, 51*, 140–148.

Toto, R. D. (2008). How to launch a successful career in clinical research: Tips on making the most of available resources. *Journal of Investigative Medicine, 56*(6), 843–846.

Varcoe, C., Hankivsky, O., Ford-Gilboe, M., Wuest, J., Wilk, P., & Campbell, J. C. (2011). Attributing selected costs to intimate partner violence in a sample of women who have left abusive partners: A social determinant of health approach. *Canadian Public Policy, 37*, 359–380.

Wenger, E. (1998). *Communities of practice: Learning, meaning, and identity*. Cambridge, UK: Cambridge University Press.

West, M. A. (1994). *Effective teamwork*. Leicester, UK: BPS Books.

Whittemore, R. (2007). Top 10 tips for beginning a program of research. *Research in Nursing & Health, 30*, 235–237.

Wuest, J., Ford-Gilboe, M., Merritt-Gray, M., & Berman, H. (2003). Intrusion: The central problem for family health promotion among children and single mothers after leaving an abusive partner. *Qualitative Health Research, 13*, 597–622.

Wuest, J., Ford-Gilboe, M., Merritt-Gray, M., & Varcoe, C. (2013). Building on "grab," attending to "fit," and being prepared to "modify": How grounded theory "works" to guide a health intervention for abused women. In C. T. Beck (Ed.), *Routledge international handbook of qualitative nursing research* (pp. 32–46). New York, NY: Routledge.

Wuest, J., Ford-Gilboe, M., Merritt-Gray, M., Wilk, P., Campbell, J. C., Lent, B., Varcoe, C., & Smye, V. (2010). Pathways of chronic pain in survivors of intimate partner violence. *Journal of Women's Health, 19*(9), 1665–1674.

Wuest, J., & Hodgins, M. J. (2011). Reflections on methodological approaches and conceptual contributions on a program of caregiving research: Development and testing of Wuest's theory of family caregiving. *Qualitative Health Research, 21*(2), 151–161.

Wuest, J., & Merritt-Gray, M. (1999). Not going back: Sustaining the separation in the process of leaving abusive relationships. *Violence Against Women, 5*, 110–133.

S • I • X

Other Nurse Researchers' Programs of Research

As a single footstep will not make a path on the earth,
so a single thought will not make a pathway in
the mind. To make a deep physical path, we
walk again and again. To make a deep mental
path, we must think over and over the kind of
thoughts we wish to dominate our lives.

—*Henry David Thoreau*

PAMELA HINDS'S PROGRAM OF RESEARCH IN PEDIATRIC ONCOLOGY

Back in the 1990s when Hinds began her research program on fatigue in children and adolescents with cancer, she noted that extensive research had been conducted on fatigue in adults with cancer but not in children. Hinds and her colleague Hockenberry-Eaton (2000) believed that this lack of attention to fatigue in children and adolescents with cancer was due to a number of reasons:

- Dose-limiting parameters do not address fatigue as a side effect in children
- Children do not actively communicate their concerns regarding oncology treatment side effects
- Parents are not aware that their child's fatigue is a side effect that warrants intervention

From their clinical experience, Hockenberry-Eaton and Hinds (2000) shared a typical case study illustrating a child's fatigue while undergoing cancer treatment:

> Johnny is a 10-year-old with T-cell lymphoma who is presently receiving chemotherapy. He describes how active and playful he was before his diagnosis. Since he started treatment, he is less active, frequently complains of weakness and feeling tired, and only wants to lie around. He is unable to participate in sports like baseball because he finds it hard to run like he used to. He is often unable to attend school because he needs so much assistance and is frequently too tired to concentrate on his work. Johnny reports that resting during the day sometimes can relieve the tiredness he feels so often. He also feels mad and sad sometimes because he is too tired to play with his friends. (pp. 261–262)

In 1996, Hockenberry-Eaton and Hinds were awarded a Fatigue Clinical Scholars Research grant by the Oncology Nursing Foundation and Ortho-Biotech Corporation for the purpose of developing a program of research focusing on fatigue in children and adolescents with cancer. These nurse researchers identified four assumptions based on their clinical experiences to guide their developing research trajectory:

1. Fatigue exists in children and adolescents who are receiving treatment for cancer.
2. Fatigue in this population is a functionally limiting symptom that, if better understood, could be more accurately and completely assessed.
3. Understanding fatigue in this population means considering human development and maturation in the context of active treatment.
4. Understanding fatigue in this population will be more complete if the perspectives of the patient, parents, and staff are made visible. (Hockenberry-Eaton & Hinds, 2000, p. 262)

In the first study in Hinds's research program on fatigue in children and adolescents diagnosed with cancer, she developed conceptual and operational definitions of fatigue in this population from the perspectives of the child, parents, and staff. Contributing factors and alleviating factors that influenced pediatric oncology patients' fatigue were also identified. Patient, parent, and staff self-report instruments were developed to measure fatigue. Two factors contributing to fatigue that were identified most frequently by all three groups were anemia and lack of sleep. Hinds chose these two factors to study next in her research trajectory not only because they were listed with greater frequency, but also because they could be amenable to patient care interventions to be designed later in her research program.

Next in her program of research, Hinds conducted two observational projects. The aim of one of the projects was to examine the amount of time pediatric oncology inpatients spent during the day on various activities, such as watching TV, napping, and interacting with family and staff. In the second study, Hinds observed the number of times both staff and family members went into the child's hospital room during the night time shift, and recorded how much time was spent in the room. Hinds's thinking behind these two studies was that the data would help her research team design interventions to decrease sleep disruption and indirectly decrease the child's fatigue. At this time in her research trajectory, Hinds was planning a study to measure the relationship between anemia, a pharmacologic intervention, and fatigue in newly diagnosed children with cancer.

In one part of her research program, Hinds shared the valuable benefits of conducting a pilot feasibility study. In 2007, Hinds and her research team conducted a feasibility study of an enhanced physical activity intervention in hospitalized children and adolescents receiving chemotherapy for cancer. The intervention of pedaling a stationary bicycle-style exerciser for 30 minutes twice a day for 2 to 4 days of hospitalization was tested with a prospective, two-site randomized controlled pilot study. Hinds et al. (2007) reported that this pilot study yielded important information on the feasibility of delivering this intervention in hospitalized oncology patients. One of the important findings focused on statistical approaches to measure symptom change over time. The research team found that averaging the variable scores across data collection points lacked sensitivity to change. In a future full efficacy study, differences in sleep will be examined between the baseline symptom score and the score of each subsequent day. Averaging scores diluted the variations in sleep experienced by oncology children and adolescent patients during each day of their hospitalization. As illustrated in Table 6.1, Hinds has been a prolific researcher, developing a trajectory that was knowledge driven and not method limited.

JOANNE HALL'S PROGRAM OF RESEARCH WITH MARGINALIZED GROUPS

Hall's qualitative program of research provides a window on trauma experiences in marginalized groups. She began her research trajectory in her dissertation work, where she explored lesbians' experiences of recovery from alcohol problems using critical ethnography. Almost half of Hall's sample shared that they were survivors of child sexual abuse. This unexpected finding led Hall down the path of the second study in her research program, where her sample comprised African American women child sexual abuse

• **TABLE 6.1** Hinds's Program of Research Using Both Qualitative and Quantitative Methods

Qualitative Research	Quantitative Research
	1992 APON Delphi study to establish research priorities for pediatric oncology patients (Hinds et al., 1994)
Decision making by parents and healthcare professionals when considering continued care for pediatric patients with cancer (Hinds et al., 1997)	
Comparing patient, parent and staff descriptions of fatigue in pediatric oncology (Hinds et al., 1999)	
International feasibility study of parental decision making in pediatric oncology (Hinds et al., 2000)	
Quality of life conveyed by pediatric patients with cancer (Hinds et al., 2004)	
End of life care preferences of pediatric patients with cancer (Hinds et al., 2005a)	Hemoglobin response and improvements in quality of life in anemic children with cancer receiving myelosuppressive chemotherapy (Hinds et al., 2005b)
	Clinical field testing of an enhanced activity intervention in hospitalized children with cancer (Hinds et al., 2007a)
	Nocturnal awakenings, sleep environment interruptions and fatigue in hospitalized children with cancer (Hinds et al., 2007b)
"Trying to be a good parent" as defined by interviews with parents who made phase 1, terminal care and resuscitation decisions for their children (Hinds et al., 2009b)	Aggressive treatment of non-metastatic osteosarcoma improves health-related quality of life in children and adolescents (Hinds et al., 2009c)

(continued)

• TABLE 6.1 Hinds's Program of Research Using Both Qualitative and Quantitative Methods (*continued*)

Qualitative Research	Quantitative Research
	Health-related quality of life in adolescents at the time of diagnosis with osteosarcoma or acute myeloid leukemia (Hinds et al., 2009a)
	Psychometric and clinical assessment of the 10-item reduced version of the Fatigue Scale-Child instrument (Hinds et al., 2010)
	Parent-clinician communication intervention during end-of-life decision making for children with incurable cancer (Hinds et al., 2012)
	PROMIS pediatric measures in pediatric oncology: Valid and clinically feasible indicators of patient-reported outcomes (Hinds et al., 2013)

survivors in the beginning stages of substance recovery (Hall, 2013). The centrality of trauma in the lives of recovering women abuse survivors was becoming evident to Hall. As a result of what Hall was learning from the participants in her qualitative studies, she broadened her research to include women regardless of their sexual orientation or type of childhood maltreatment. Hall (2013) shared her rationale for her choice of qualitative research:

> A survey would not have been attractive to any of the women in exposing their marginalization, addiction and violent victimization. When the idea the participant wants to express is not in the instrument, a message is delivered that one's experience is "not on the map." This invalidation leads to mistrust and avoidance not only of research but of health care. In personal stories, socio-political-cultural context and subjective uniqueness resonate. Additionally, the use of narrative can detail the intersections of gender, race, sexual orientation, gender identity, and other sources of marginalization. (p. 49)

In reviewing transcripts, Hall noted that there was a focus on sexual abuse, to the exclusion of other forms of maltreatment after one participant asked, "Why is it only incest and sexual abuse that you are interested in? Why is it okay to beat your children?" Looking into some statistics, Hall also noted that the most common form of maltreatment was, in fact, neglect. Thus, she opened future studies to women surviving all forms of maltreatment—physical, sexual, and verbal abuse—as well as neglect. This revealed how two or more forms of maltreatment were often present for these women.

In reviewing the literature prior to the start of another study in her trauma research program, Hall et al. (2009) identified a gap in the literature. "What is missing from this newer and more hopeful literature is the explanation of how some individuals survive, and even begin to thrive. This gap motivated the present qualitative study. Our study sought to identify 'what worked' from the first-person perspective of adult female abuse survivors" (p. 376). Hall and colleagues used a feminist interpretive design in this research.

Hall (2011) also used narrative methods to study trauma recovery from childhood maltreatment. She put together an interdisciplinary team representing the disciplines of nursing, psychology, psychiatry, and women's studies. The focus of this constructivist, feminist, narrative study was the success or thriving of women who survived childhood maltreatment. Analysis of the narratives revealed a trauma recovery process called "becoming resolute." Subanalyses concentrated on key relationships, life trajectories, self-strategies, and perceptual changes.

Hall (2013) stressed to researchers that merely using a qualitative research approach does not assure you of experiential validation. Your interview questions may, in actuality, invalidate the experience a researcher is exploring. The interview questions should not be just reiterating the research questions. The language and sequence of the interview questions should encourage participants to share the "edges" of their experiences. To illustrate this point for future qualitative researchers, Hall (2013) shared the following example:

> The question "What is it like to be an abuse survivor?" might invalidate many Appalachian women, who do not use the terms "abuse" or "survivor." "How have you become successful?" may alienate those who do not feel successful. . . . Thus in approaching the topic obliquely versus head on, we asked, "What made it hard for you growing up?" (p. 49)

JANICE MORSE'S PROGRAM OF RESEARCH ON SUFFERING

Morse (2002) stressed that for researchers to fully understand complex human phenomena, such as suffering, triangulation of results from multiple separate research studies using diverse qualitative methods is required. Morse reported that there existed a huge methodological gap in the literature regarding suffering. Researchers were focusing on narratives of suffering but ignoring observations of patients who were suffering. Observational research supplements interviews and yields different information that complements interview data. The behavior of the sufferer is illuminated through different levels of analysis and various foci. Morse conducted studies using interviews, narratives, and participant observation. Through these multiple methods of qualitative research, Morse developed a model of suffering that displayed the relationship between the two states, the emotionless state of enduring and the state of emotional suffering. Morse's model of suffering then became the framework for future studies in her program of research.

At this stage in her research trajectory, Morse realized that participant observation of suffering in trauma was not an adequate method. She instituted videotaping, which allowed the use of approaches related to microanalytic analysis, such as qualitative ethology and linguistic analysis. With the help of videotapes, Morse examined the interactions between family members, the patient, and the caregivers. Morse used eight different methods to examine the various dimensions of suffering in her early work in her research program (Table 6.2).

In 2001, Morse developed a Praxis Theory of Suffering based on the major findings from her program of research to date on the behavioral–experiential nature of suffering. In this theory, suffering is viewed as consisting of two major behavioral states: (a) enduring, in which emotions are suppressed and (b) emotional suffering, in which emotions are released in an overt state of distress (Figure 6.1).

Continuing in her program of research, Morse, Beres, Spiers, Mayan, and Olson (2003) described facial expressions of enduring and emotional suffering in order to link them with verbal narrative. They used Ekman and Friesen's (1978) facial action coding system. As a result of this innovative study, Morse and colleagues were able to microanalytically examine the two behavioral states in suffering so that in future research, appropriate comforting responses can be identified to help relieve suffering.

The most recent version of Morse's Praxis Theory of Suffering (Morse, 2010) includes her synthesis of three decades of qualitative studies (Table 6.3). In this table, one can see her exemplary systematic program of research. Morse stated that the real value of her research on suffering is that through observation of suffering behaviors, facial expressions, and interactions, nurses can immediately recognize suffering and immediately interact appropriately with patients in crisis and intervene. Morse hopes that the real change her program of research will have is a decreased reliance on formal assessment and an increased ability to instantly recognize our patients' suffering and

• TABLE 6.2 Studies in Morse's Early Research Program Pertaining to Suffering, Major Findings, Methods Used, and References

Topic	Project	Major Findings	Research Method	References
Illness experience	Suffering trajectory of patients and families with various conditions	Illness constellation model	Grounded theory	Morse and Johnson (1991)
Accident experience	Suffering trajectory from victim to patient to disabled person	Model of preserving self	Grounded theory	Morse and O'Brien (1995)
Comfort	Meaning of discomfort and modes of seeking comfort	The fundamental experience of illness was that of suffering	Phenomenology	Morse, Bottorff, and Hutchinson (1994, 1995)
	Experience of shared pain	Identification and description of compathy	Concept identification	Morse and Mitcham (1997); Morse, Mitcham, and van der Steen (1998)
Trauma care	Observed how nurses comforted patients when analgesics were delayed or withheld	Comfort talk register Identified states of enduring	Nonparticipant observations/video/ linguistic analysis	Proctor, Morse, and Khonsari (1996); Morse and Proctor (1998)
Suffering	Delineated the states of suffering and enduring	Model of suffering	Concept identification	Morse and Carter (1996)
	Interviews with burn patients	Applied concept to individual experience	Grounded theory	Morse and Carter (1995)

(continued)

• TABLE 6.2 Studies in Morse's Early Research Program Pertaining to Suffering, Major Findings, Methods Used, and References (continued)

Topic	Project	Major Findings	Research Method	References
Enduring to die	Interviews with patients who had been informed that "nothing more could be done" medically	Linked trajectories of the illness experience and dying	Grounded theory	Olson, Morse, Smith, Mayan, and Hammond (2001)
	Videotaped interviews with those who had suffered or their relatives	Identified cocooning Explores the transition between enduring and emotionally suffering	Qualitative ethology and conversational analysis	Morse, Beres, Spiers, Mayan, and Olson (2003)
Suffering of relatives	Observation of relatives as they entered the trauma room	Synchrony of suffering Sideswiping	Video/qualitative ethology	Morse and Pooler (2002)
Developing theory of suffering	Integration of all studies	Project triangulation	Developing qualitatively derived theory	Morse (2001)
	Examination of relationship of hope with releasing	Linking allied concepts		Morse and Penrod (1999)
Responding to suffering	Revisiting comforting of the sufferer	Comforting interaction model Analysis of caregiver responses to the sufferer	Theoretical synthesis of the studies	Morse, Havens, and Wilson (1997); Morse (2000)
Application	Examination of nasogastric tube insertion using suffering/comforting model	Identified and compared caregiver styles, effectiveness of nasogastric tube insertion	Qualitative ethology	Morse, Penrod, Kassab, and Dellasega (2000); Penrod, Morse, and Wilson (1999)

Reprinted with permission from Morse (2002, p. 126).

• **FIGURE 6.1 Model of Suffering**

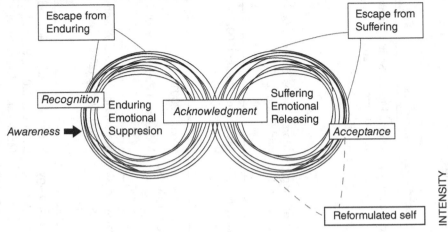

Reprinted with permission from Morse (2001, p. 54).

administer immediate behavioral assessment strategies (Morse, personal communication, 2014).

KARIN OLSON'S PROGRAM OF RESEARCH ON FATIGUE

After Olson completed her first study on fatigue using grounded theory, she reviewed the current state of the literature before deciding on her next research project. She found that the definition of fatigue being used in most nursing research was incomplete when she compared it with the findings from her qualitative research. Olson decided that the next study in her program of research would focus on reconceptualizing fatigue. Her aim was to find a common core set of characteristics of fatigue across groups who experience fatigue for various reasons. Using the pragmatic utility approach for concept analysis that is based on published data, Olson reviewed qualitative studies conducted on fatigue in shift workers, athletes, persons with chronic fatigue syndrome, depression, or cancer (Olson & Morse, 2005). This concept analysis revealed six common characteristics of fatigue across these five study groups: muscular changes, cognitive changes, sleep disturbance, emotional changes, social disruption, and body sensation changes.

The next five subsequent studies in Olson's program of research sought to validate the results of her concept analysis of fatigue. One study was conducted with each of the five study groups included in the concept analysis.

• TABLE 6.3 Research for the Development of Morse's Praxis Theory of Suffering: Components, Progress, and Funding Received

1. Background (1985–1991)
Goal: To develop grounded theories of illness experience/trajectory of suffering: e.g., trajectories of myocardial infarction, hysterectomy, discharge from psychiatric hospital, adolescent abortion, impact of chemotherapy on the family
Funding: Small grants
Metasynthesis: The illness experience: dimensions of suffering
⬇
2. Delineation of comfort and comforting (1991–1994)
Goal: To delineate the concepts inherent in comforting
Concepts: Caring, empathy, trust, social support, reciprocity, compathy, patterns of touch (infants)
Funding: NRC NIH R01 (3-year foreign award)
⬇
3. Identification of role of suffering in comforting (1994–1996)
Goal: Identification of role of suffering in comforting
Strategies: Comfort talk register, nasogastric tube insertion, family presence in trauma care, pain dialogues, normalization
Funding: NINR NIH R01 continuation grant (5 years)
⬇
4. Explication of suffering behaviors (1997–2001)
Goal: Development of praxis theory of suffering
Model of "preserving self," development of praxis theory of suffering, model of reformulated self
Funding: NINR NIH R01 (continuation)
⬇
5. Identification of patterns of suffering (2001–2006)
Identification of patterns of suffering and further development of the praxis theory of suffering facial coding system for expressions of suffering, synchrony of suffering, patterns of suffering during breast cancer diagnosis
Funding: CIHR, Canadian Breast CA FDN
⬇
6. Anticipated outcomes of this application (2010–2015)
Verified theory
Compendium of enduring behaviors
Clinical implementation model

Reprinted with permission from Morse (2010, p. 571).

Ethnoscience and grounded theory were the qualitative methods used to tease out manifestations of and differences among fatigue, tiredness, and exhaustion.

Armed with their conceptual definitions of fatigue and two related concepts, Olson's research team next constructed a conceptual framework of the relationships of these three concepts that could be used to develop interventions for fatigue. The Revised Edmonton Fatigue Framework is the current configuration of Olson's conceptual framework, in which the primary propositions are as follows:

1. Adaptive capacity is a function of nutrition, cognition, muscle endurance, sleep, social interaction, emotional reactivity, demographic factors (disease state, age, and gender), other symptoms, and the social context within which these elements occur.
2. Adaptive capacity is inversely related to allostatic overload and fatigue. As adaptive capacity increases, allostatic overload and fatigue decline. (Olson, 2013, p. 69)

Because the concept of adaptive capacity was a somewhat new concept, Olson's next study in her research trajectory led her down the path to operationalize it. This step required instrument development of the Adaptive Capacity Index (Olson et al., 2011). Olson's rationale behind this instrument development was to have a scale that would allow her research team to test hypotheses regarding adaptive capacity and allostatic loading.

Olson and her research team began to think more about fatigue in the context of symptom clusters. In her model, this point is represented by "other symptoms." Olson wanted to figure out how all the pieces went together in her model of fatigue. Other symptoms frequently drive fatigue, and she wanted to know how they were related. At this point, Olson audited a course in structural equation modeling. The primary analytic approach at this time was factor analysis. Olson, who has a PhD in educational psychology with a focus in measurement, was concerned that researchers using factor analysis to study symptom clusters did not have a full appreciation of its assumptions and thus their interpretations of their results may not be valid (Olson, personal communication, February 1, 2014). The local palliative care program had a large database that consisted of symptom scores over time for palliative patients. Olson and her research team extracted cases from this database that had data at two points in time close to the end of life. The hypothesis that Olson wanted to test with structural equation modeling was that contrary to work published to date, symptom clusters were not stable. The relationships among symptoms changed over time. Olson's research supported this hypothesis (Hayduk, Olson, Quan, Cree, & Cui, 2010; Olson et al., 2008).

Next, Olson decided to reanalyze the same data set using factor analysis to show that the results were not the same. An interesting part of her findings was that when the assumptions of factor analysis were kept in mind, the findings from the factor analysis were essentially uninterpretable and did not fit her team's clinical experience (Olson, Hayduk, & Thomas, 2014). Olson's take-home message for graduate students thinking of developing a program of research is that decisions regarding design and analysis require a thorough working knowledge of the underlying assumptions of both (Olson, personal communication, February 1, 2014).

At this fork in the road of her research program, Olson realized she needed to expand her research team to include some colleagues in the biological sciences since she would now be studying adaptive capacity and allostatic loading. Adding scientists in the biological field would help to link the biological and psychosocial components of her fatigue framework. Currently, her research team includes physicians and individuals with PhDs in immunology, psychology, physiology, and biochemistry, in addition to nurse researchers.

Olson's research team is currently examining different social contexts that can impact the meaning of fatigue. Up to this time, Olson's studies had been conducted in Canada, so now the next path in her research trajectory is leading her to investigate the meaning of fatigue related to geography. Cancer-related fatigue in the following five countries is being studied: Thailand, Italy, England, Sweden, and Canada (Graffigna, Vegni, Barello, Olson, & Bosio, 2011; Kirshbaum, Olson, Pongthavornkamol, & Graffigna, 2013; Pongthavornkamol et al., 2012). Olson chose ethnoscience at this stage in her research program in order to study language as a way to uncover beliefs and values that shape the meaning of fatigue. In ethnoscience, the focus is on identifying not themes but key words and phrases, in this case regarding the experience of fatigue, and then determining how these words and phrases are related to each other.

Olson was fortunate to have a personnel award from the Alberta Heritage Foundation for Medical Research (now Alberta Innovates Health Solutions). As a result, Olson taught only one course per year for 7 years, which allowed her to do all this work on her research program.

RUTH McCORKLE'S PROGRAM OF RESEARCH IN ONCOLOGY

Early in her research career, McCorkle was taught the importance of documenting any problems she was having in her day-to-day research operations and to share these with other researchers. McCorkle (2011) shared some of the lessons she learned in the day-to-day operations of her program of research in some of her publications (Table 6.4). As she stated, "[T]hese lessons learned can be incredibly helpful to others and facilitate their research as they start on a similar path" (p. 336).

At the 30-year mark of her research program on patient and caregiver outcomes in cancer care, McCorkle (2006) described its three-phase evolution to that date. Phase 1 focused on instrument development. In 1976, McCorkle

• **TABLE 6.4 Examples of McCorkle's Contributions to the Research Process**

Author (Year)	Study	Citation
McCorkle and Young (1978)	Development of a Symptom Distress Scale	*Cancer Nursing, 1*(5), 373–378
McCorkle et al. (1984)	Subject accrual and attention: Problems and solutions	*Journal of Psychosocial Oncology, 2*(3/4), 137–146
McCorkle (1987)	The measurement of symptom distress	*Seminars in Oncology Nursing, 3,* 234–256
Lowery and McCorkle (1991)	Advanced care in serious illness: Evolution of a center	*Journal of Professional Nursing, 7*(3), 152–159
Lev et al. (1993)	A shortened version of an instrument measuring bereavement	*International Journal of Nursing Studies, 30*(3), 213–226
Bang et al. (1994)	Development of a self-administrated psychosocial cancer screening tool	*Cancer Practice, 2*(4), 288–296
Norman et al. (2001)	Development and validation of a telephone questionnaire to measure lymphedema in women treated for breast cancer	*Physical Therapy, 81*(6), 1192–1205
Tang and McCorkle (2002)	Appropriate time frame for data collection in quality of life research among cancer patients at the end of life	*Quality of Life Research, 11*(2), 145–155
Tang and McCorkle (2002)	Use of family proxies in quality of life research for cancer patients at the end of life: A literature review	*Cancer Investigation, 20*(7&8), 1086–1104
Cooley et al. (2004)	Comparison of health-related quality of life questionnaires in ambulatory oncology	*Quality of Life Research, 14*(15), 1–11
Robinson et al. (2007)	Psychometric properties of the Male Urogenital Distress Inventory (MUDI) and Male Urinary Symptom Impact Questionnaire (MUSIQ) in radical prostatectomy patients	*Urologic Nursing, 27*(6), 512–518

(continued)

• TABLE 6.4 Examples of McCorkle's Contributions to the Research Process (*continued*)

Author (Year)	Study	Citation
Jenerette et al. (2008)	Models of inter-institutional collaboration to build research capacity for reducing health disparities	*Nursing Outlook,* 56(1), 16–24
McCorkle (2011)	Interdisciplinary collaboration in the pursuit of science to improve psychosocial cancer care	*Psycho-Oncology,* 20(5), 538–543
Cohen et al. (2011)	Lessons learned in research collaborations and dissemination in a National Institute of Nursing Research-Funded Research Center	*Journal of Professional Nursing, 27*(3), 153–160
Lazenby et al. (2012)	Validity of the end-of-life professional caregiver survey to assess for multidisciplinary educational needs	*Journal of Palliative Medicine, 15*(4), 427–431

and her research team discovered that reliable and valid instruments to measure the outcomes of symptom distress and functional status were not available. As a result, her research path took an unexpected turn toward instrument development and psychometric testing. Next, armed with her psychometrically sound instruments, McCorkle embarked on Phase 2 of her research trajectory, which focused on testing the effects of the impact of the role of advanced practice nursing on interventions to decrease cancer treatment–related symptoms and increase functional abilities. Translation methods took center stage in Phase 3. During this phase, McCorkle's patient and caregiver studies influenced changes in policy and practice. For example, her study on the impact of home care, funded by the National Center for Nursing Research and the National Cancer Institute, impacted the 1992 Family Leave Bill.

REFERENCES

Ekman, P., & Friesen, W. V. (1978). *Facial action coding system: A technique for measurement of facial movement.* Palto Alto, CA: Consulting Psychologists Press.

Graffigna, G., Vegni, E., Barello, S., Olson, K., & Bosio, C. A. (2011). Studying the social construction of cancer–related fatigue: The heuristic value to ethnoscience. *Patient Education and Counseling, 82,* 402–409.

Hall, J. M. (2011). Narrative methods in a study of trauma recovery. *Qualitative Health Research, 21*(1), 3–13.

Hall, J. M. (2013). The power of qualitative inquiry: Traumatic experiences of marginalized groups. In C. T. Beck (Ed.), *Routledge international handbook of qualitative nursing research* (pp. 47–63). New York, NY: Routledge.

Hall, J. M., Roman, M. W., Thomas, S. P., Travis, C. B., Powell, J., Tennison, C. R., . . . McArthur, P. M. (2009). Thriving is becoming resolute in narratives of women surviving childhood maltreatment. *American Journal of Orthopsychiatry, 79*(3), 375–386.

Hayduk, L., Olson, K., Quan, H., Cree, M., & Cui, Y. (2010). Temporal changes in the causal foundations of palliative care symptoms. *Quality of Life Research, 19*(3), 299–306.

Hinds, P. S., Billups, C. A., Cao, X., Gattuso, J. S., Burghen, E., West, N. . . . Daw, N. C. (2009a). Health-related quality of life in adolescents at the time of diagnosis with osteosarcoma or acute myeloid leukemia. *European Journal of Oncology Nursing, 13*, 156–163.

Hinds, P. S., Drew, D., Oakes, L. L., Fouladi, M., Spunt, S. L., Church, C., & Furman, W. L. (2005a). End-of-life care preferences of pediatric patients with cancer. *Journal of Clinical Oncology, 23*(36), 9146–9154.

Hinds, P. S., Gattuso, J. S., Billups, C. A., West, N. K., Wu, J., Rivera, C., . . . Daw, N. C. (2009c). Aggressive treatment of non-metastatic osteosarcoma improves health-related quality of life in children and adolescents. *European Journal of Cancer, 45*, 2007–2014.

Hinds, P. S., Gattuso, J. S., Fletcher, A., Baker, E., Coleman, B., Jackson, T., . . . Pui, C. H. (2004). Quality of life as conveyed by pediatric patients. *Quality of Life Research, 13*, 761–772.

Hinds, P. S., Hockenberry-Eaton, M., Feusner, J., Hord, J. D., Rackoff, W., & Rozzouk, B. (2005b). Hemoglobin response and improvements in quality of life in anemic children with cancer receiving myelosuppressive chemotherapy. *The Journal of Supportive Oncology, 3*(6, Suppl. 4), 10–11.

Hinds, P. S., Hockenberry-Eaton, M., Gilger, E., Kline, N., Burleson, C., Bottomley, S., & Quargnenti, A. (1999). Comparing patient, parent, and staff descriptions of fatigue in pediatric oncology patients. *Cancer Nursing, 22*; 277–289.

Hinds, P. S., Hockenberry-Eaton, M., Rai, S. N., Zhang, L., Razzouk, B. I., Cremer, L., . . . Rodriguez–Galindo, C. (2007a). Clinical field testing of an enhanced–activity intervention in hospitalized children with cancer. *Journal of Pain and Symptom Management, 33*(6), 686–697.

Hinds, P. S., Hockenberry-Eaton. M., Rai, S. N., Zhang, L., Razzouk, B. I., McCarthy, K., . . . Rodriguez Galindo, C. (2007b). Noctural awakenings, sleep environment interruptions, and fatigue in hospitalized children with cancer. *Oncology Nursing Forum, 34*(2), 393–402.

Hinds, P. S., Nuss, S. L., Ruccione, K. S., Withycombe, J. S., Jacobs, S., DeLuca, H., . . . DeWatt, D. A. (2013). PROMIS pediatric measures in pediatric oncology: Valid and clinically feasible indictors of patient reported outcomes. *Pediatric Blood Cancer, 60*, 402–408.

Hinds, P. S., Quargnenti, A., Olson, M. S., Gross, J., Puckett, P., Randall, E., . . . Wiedenhoffer, D. (1994). The 1992 APON Delphi study to establish research priorities for pediatric oncology nursing. *Journal of Pediatric Oncology Nursing, 11*(1), 20–27.

Hinds, P. S., Oakes, L., Furman, W., Foppiano, P., Olson, M. S., Quargnenti, A., . . . Strong, C. (1997). Decision making by parents and healthcare professionals when considering continued care for pediatric patients with cancer. *Oncology Nursing Forum, 24*, 1523–1528.

Hinds, P. S., Oakes, L. L., Hicks, J., Powell, B., Srivastava, D. K., Spunt, S. L., . . . Furman, W. L. (2009b). "Trying to be a good parent" as defined by interviews with parents who made phase 1, terminal care, and resuscitation decisions for their children. *Journal of Clinical Oncology, 27*(35), 5979–5985.

Hinds, P. S., Oakes, L. L., Hicks, J., Powell, B., Srivastava, D. K., Baker, J. N., . . . Furman, W. L. (2012). Parent-clinician communication intervention during end-of-life decision making for children with incurable cancer. *Journal of Palliative Medicine, 15*(8), 916–922.

Hinds, P. S., Oakes, L., Quargnenti, A., Furman, W., Bowman, L., Gilger, E., . . . Drew, D. (2000). An international feasibility study of parental decision making in pediatric oncology. *Oncology Nursing Forum, 27*(8), 1233–1243.

Hinds, P. S., Yang, J., Gattuso, J. S., Hockenberry-Eaton, M., Jones, H., Zupanec, S., . . . Srivastava, D. K. (2010). Psychometric and clinical assessment of the 10-item reduced version of the Fatigue Scale–Child Instrument. *Journal of Pain and Symptom Management, 39*(3), 572–578.

Hockenberry-Eaton, M., & Hinds, P. S. (2000). Fatigue in children and adolescents with cancer: Evolution of a program of study. *Seminars in Oncology Nursing, 16*(4), 261–272.

Kirshbaum, M. N., Olson, K., Pongthavornkamol, K., & Graffigna, G. (2013). Understanding the meaning of fatigue at the end of life: An ethnoscience approach. *European Journal of Oncology Nursing, 17,* 146–153.

McCorkle, R. (2006). A program of research on patient and family caregiver outcomes: Three phases of evolution. *Oncology Nursing Forum, 33*(1), 25–31.

McCorkle, R. (2011). A purposeful career path to make a difference in cancer care. *Cancer Nursing, 34*(4), 335–339.

Morse, J. M. (2000). On comfort and comforting. *America Journal of Nursing, 100*(9), 34–38.

Morse, J. M. (2001). Toward a praxis theory of suffering. *Advances in Nursing Science, 24*(1), 47–59.

Morse, J. M. (2002). Qualitative health research: Challenges for the 21st century. *Qualitative Health Research, 12*(1), 116–129.

Morse, J. M. (2010). The Praxis theory of suffering. In J. B. Butts & K. L. Rich (Eds.), *Philosophies and theories in advanced nursing practice* (pp. 569–602). Sudbury, MA: Jones & Bartlett.

Morse, J. M., Beres, M. A., Spiers, J. A., Mayan, M., & Olson, K. (2003). Identifying signals of suffering by linking verbal and facial cues. *Qualitative Health Research, 13*(8), 1063– 1077.

Morse, J. M., Bottorff, J. L., & Hutchinson, S. (1994). The phenomenology of comfort. *Journal of Advanced Nursing, 20,* 189–195.

Morse, J. M., Bottorff, J. L., & Hutchinson, S. (1995). The paradox of comfort. *Nursing Research, 44* (1), 14–19.

Morse, J. M., & Carter, B. J. (1995). Strategies of enduring and the suffering of loss: Modes of comfort used by a resilient survivor. *Holistic Nursing Practice, 9*(3), 33–58.

Morse, J. M., & Carter, B. J. (1996). The essence of enduring and the expression of suffering: The reformulation of self. *Scholarly Inquiry for Nursing Practice, 10*(1), 43–60.

Morse, J. M., Havens, G. A., & Wilson, S. (1997). The comforting interaction: Developing a model of nurse–patient relationship. *Scholarly Inquiry for Nursing Practice, 11*(4), 321– 347.

Morse, J. M., & Johnson, J. L. (1991). Towards a theory of illness, In J. M. Morse & J. L. Johnson (Eds.), *Understanding the illness experience: Dimensions of suffering* (pp. 315–342). Newbury Park, CA: SAGE.

Morse, J. M., & Mitcham, C. (1997). Compathy: The contagion of physical distress. *Journal of Advanced Nursing, 26,* 649–657.

Morse, J. M., & O'Brien, B. (1995). Preserving self: From victim, to patient, to disabled person. *Journal of Advanced Nursing, 21,* 886–896.

Morse, J. M., & Penrod, J. (1999). Linking concepts of enduring, suffering, and hope. *Image: Journal of Nursing Scholarship, 31*(2), 145–150.

Morse, J. M., & Pooler, C. (2002). Patient-family–nurse interactions in the trauma resuscitation room. *American Journal of Critical Care, 11*(3), 240–249.

Morse, J. M., & Proctor, A. (1998). Maintaining patient endurance: The comfort work of trauma nurses. *Clinical Nursing Research, 7*(3), 250–274.

Morse, J. M., Mitcham, C., & van der Steen, V. (1998). Compathy or physical empathy: Implications for the caregiver relationship. *Journal of Medical Humanities, 19*(1), 51–65.

Morse, J. M., Penrod, J., Kassab, C., & Dellasega, C. (2000). Evaluating the efficiency and effectiveness of approaches to nasogastric tub insertion during trauma care. *American Journal of Critical Care, 9*(5), 325–333.

Olson, K. (2013). Learning about the nature of fatigue. In C. T. Beck (Ed.), *Routledge international handbook of qualitative nursing research* (pp. 64–74). New York, NY: Routledge.

Olson, K., Hayduk, L., Cree, M., Tsui, Y., Quan, H., Hanson, J., . . . Strasser, F. (2008). The changing causal foundations of variations in cancer–related symptom clustering during the final month of palliative care: A longitudinal study. *BMC Medical Research Methodology, 8,* 36.

Olson, K., Hayduk, L., & Thomas, J. (2014). Comparing two approaches for studying symptom clusters: Factor analysis and structural equation modeling. *Supportive Care in Cancer, 22,* 153–161.

Olson, K., & Morse, J. M. (2005). Delineating the concept of fatigue using a pragmatic utility approach. In J. Cutcliffe & H. McKenna (Eds.), *The essential concepts of nursing* (pp. 141–159). Edinburgh, UK: Elsevier.

Olson, K., Morse, J. M., Smith, J., Mayan, M., & Hammond, D. (2001). Linking trajectories of illness and dying. *Omega-Journal of Death & Dying, 42*(4), 293–308.

Olson, K., Rogers, W. T., Cui, Y., Cree, M., Baracos, V., Rust, T., . . . Bonville, N. (2011). Measuring fatigue in advanced cancer patients by assessing adaptive capacity: An instrument development study. *International Journal of Nursing Studies, 48*(8), 986–994.

Penrod, J., Morse, J. M., & Wilson, S. (1999). Comforting strategies used during nasogastric tube insertion. *Journal of Clinical Nursing, 8,* 31–38.

Pongthavornkamol, K., Olson, K., Soparatanapaisarn, N., Chatchaisucha, S., Khamkon, A., Potaros, D., . . . Graffigna, G. (2012). Comparing the meanings of fatigue in individuals with cancer in Thailand and Canada. *Cancer Nursing, 35*(5), e1–e9.

Proctor, A., Morse, J. M., & Khonsari, E. S. (1996). Sounds of comfort in the trauma center: How nurses talk to patients in pain. *Social Sciences and Medicine, 42*(12), 1669–1680.

S·E·V·E·N

Publishing Your Program of Research

No one saves us but ourselves. No one can and no one may.
We ourselves must walk the path.
—*Gautama Buddha*

If a program of research is to provide new discoveries for evidence-based practice, dissemination of its findings is a critical step. Sandelowski (2003) warns us that "the merits of a study (lie) in the ability of writers to persuade readers of its merits" (p. 321). There are many guidelines published already for writing up quantitative research such as the American Psychological Association's (APA) publication manual (APA, 2010), and the American Education Research Association's (AERA) guide for reporting research (AERA, 2006). For quantitative researchers, there is one format that is typically used to report findings. The results section is usually organized by the hypotheses tested, research questions investigated, or key variables studied with findings from the statistical tests discussed under each of these headings. There are typical tables that can be used to report results of specific statistical tests, such as a regression analysis. In writing up a qualitative study versus a quantitative study for publication, there are some differences that authors need to be aware of. Qualitative researchers face more of a challenge in writing up their results. There is no set format for reporting their findings. In addition, qualitative researchers need to be creative in presenting their findings to ensure their results have "grab."

QUALITATIVE RESEARCH

Before we go any further, I would like to include two quotes about writing qualitative research, to set the stage for this final chapter. The first is a quote from Van Manen (2002, pp. 3–4):

Writing is similar to reading in that we take leave of the common world that we share with others. We step out of one world, the ordinary world of daylight, and enter another, the textorium, the world of the text. In this world of shadows and darkness one traverses the landscape of language. One develops a special relation to language, a reflective relation which disturbs its taken-for-grantedness.

The second quote is from Eisner (1998, p. 89):

The "trick" in writing, often taken for granted, is to create in the public world a structure or form whose features re-present what is experienced in private. The sense of discovery and excitement . . . is not simply a set of words; it is a set of qualities, including a sense of energy that must somehow be made palpable through prose. This is what effective writers achieve.

In trying to accomplish this feat, important decisions need to be made about the amount of space given to the methodology versus the results of a qualitative study. Page limitations of the journal you are submitting to drive this choice. A mistake often made by new qualitative researchers is in giving more space in their manuscript to describing their findings to the detriment of providing important details of their methodology. Reviewers of journals may decide not to recommend the publication of a qualitative research manuscript because the methods used appear weak when in fact the methods used were strong but the author chose to omit this critical information and to provide more details of the findings.

In trying to trim down your qualitative findings for your manuscript, cutting out some of the vivid and powerful quotes you have included in your first draft is difficult. My PhD students have often said it is almost like having to choose one of your children over another. Trimming your results to make page limitations of a journal is an iterative process. It may take multiple go-arounds to make the final cuts.

To deal with space limitations for your manuscript, figures and tables are extremely helpful since these are usually not counted in the maximum number of pages allowed by journals. Figures and tables can also provide some of the "grab" needed in presenting qualitative results. Without a figure or table, the results section will be only words, paragraph after paragraph. When publishing a grounded theory study, for example, a figure of the stages or phases of your theory is extremely helpful. Figure 7.1 is an example of one such figure from my postpartum depression grounded theory of Teetering on the Edge (Beck, 1993). As readers progress through the findings, they can periodically orient themselves to just where they are in your grounded theory by checking back to your figure.

• **FIGURE 7.1 Four-Stage Process of Teetering on the Edge**

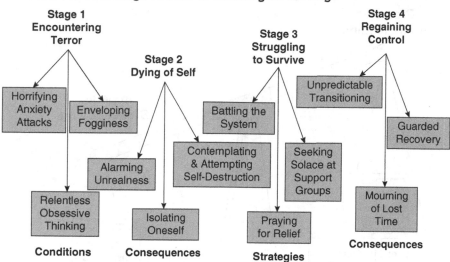

Reprinted with permission from Beck (1993, pp. 42–43).

An example of a breastfeeding scale figure I created to help display the results of the eight themes in my phenomenological study on the impact of birth trauma on breastfeeding is presented in Figure 7.2 (Beck & Watson, 2008). A second example from my research program can be found in Figure 7.3. In this figure, I added photos and images beside each of the five themes in my phenomenological study of posttraumatic stress disorder due to childbirth (Beck, 2004a). Another example of the use of a figure in one of my articles from my program of research is Figure 7.4. In this article, I included this figure I created not to illustrate my results but instead to concretely present Colaizzi's (1978) steps in his method to analyze data, which was the approach I used in that phenomenological study. A final example of the use of a figure in my program of research (Figure 7.5) was a poster of inspirational quotes one mother used in my study on subsequent childbirth following a previous birth trauma (Beck & Watson, 2010).

Use of creativity in deciding on the title of your article and the titles of your key findings, such as the themes that emerged, should not be taken lightly when writing up a qualitative study. Also, the first few sentences in your introduction beg your consideration as these are critical to hooking in the readers to your article. Examples from my phenomenological studies on traumatic childbirth are cited here to help illustrate the points I am making here. For my study on traumatic childbirth, I chose the title "Birth trauma: In the eye of the beholder" (Beck, 2004b). I started the article thus:

In her 1878 novel *Molly Bawn*, Margaret Wolfe Hungerford, an Irish-born 19th century romance novelist, first penned the phrase

- **FIGURE 7.2 Breastfeeding Scale**

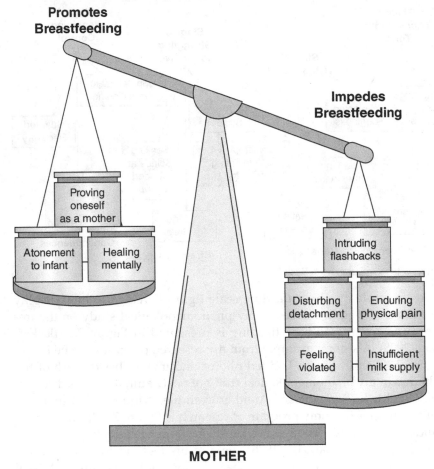

Reprinted from Beck and Watson (2008, p. 232).

"beauty is in the eye of the beholder." Beauty is not the only quality or phenomenon that lies in the eye of the beholder; birth trauma also does. What a mother perceives as birth trauma may be seen quite differently through the eyes of obstetric care providers, who may view it as a routine delivery and just another day at the hospital. (Beck, 2004b, p. 28)

The title I decided on for another study was "The anniversary of birth trauma: Failure to rescue" (Beck, 2006). For this study, I started the article off with a powerful quote from one of the mothers who participated in that study: "In the words of one mother, every birthday is no longer the celebration of the

• **FIGURE 7.3 Five Essential Themes of PTSD Due to Childbirth**

Theme #		Theme
1	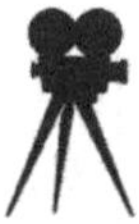	Going to the movies: Please don't make me go!
2	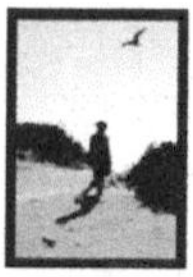	A shadow of myself: Too numb to try and change
3	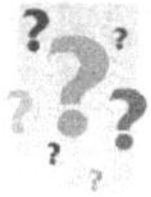	Seeking to have questions answered and wanting to talk, talk, talk
4	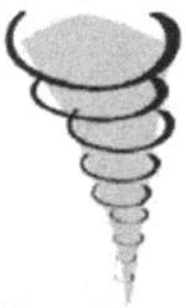	The dangerous trio of anger, anxiety, and depression: Spiraling downward
5	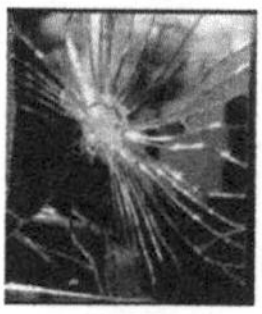	Isolation from the world of motherhood: Dreams shattered

Reprinted with permission from Beck and Watson (2008, p. 231).

child but is really an anniversary for the rape. Rape day. My son was conceived from love and born out of rape" (Beck, 2006, p. 381).

The creative titles I chose for the themes in the birth trauma study (Beck, 2004b) were:

• Theme 1: To care for me: Was that too much to ask for?
• Theme 2: To communicate with me: Why was this neglected?
• Theme 3: To provide safe care: You betrayed my trust and I felt powerless.
• Theme 4: The end justifies the means: At whose expense? At what price?

In the anniversary of birth trauma study, I chose the following titles for my themes to help bring them alive:

• Theme 1: The prologue: An agonizing time
• Theme 2: The actual day: A celebration of a birthday or the torment of an anniversary
• Theme 3: The epilogue: A fragile state
• Theme 4: Subsequent anniversaries: For better or worse

• FIGURE 7.4 Colaizzi's Procedural Steps for Analyzing Data Phenomenologically

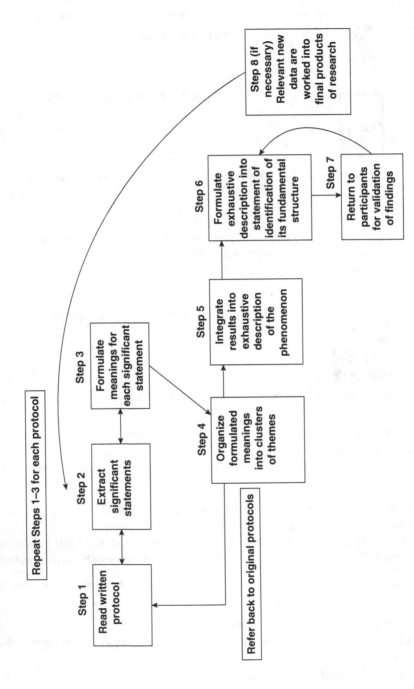

Reprinted with permission from Beck and Watson (2008, p. 231).

• **FIGURE 7.5 A Poster of Inspirational Quotes by One Mother**

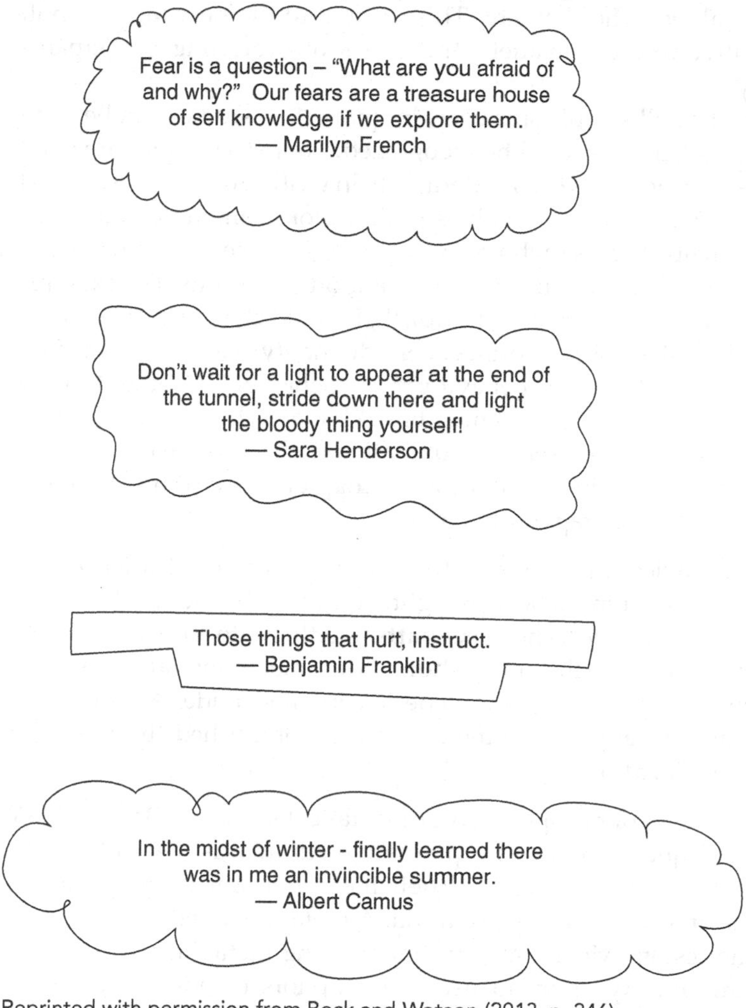

Fear is a question – "What are you afraid of and why?" Our fears are a treasure house of self knowledge if we explore them.
— Marilyn French

Don't wait for a light to appear at the end of the tunnel, stride down there and light the bloody thing yourself!
— Sara Henderson

Those things that hurt, instruct.
— Benjamin Franklin

In the midst of winter - finally learned there was in me an invincible summer.
— Albert Camus

Reprinted with permission from Beck and Watson (2013, p. 246).

Participants' quotes are often used by qualitative researchers to bring alive their findings. Sandelowski (1994) stressed the need for developing the craft of quoting. Various reasons for using quotes can include providing evidence for points being made, illustrating a concrete example, including the feelings and thoughts of participants, and evoking a response in readers to the article. Sandelowski (1994) identified the following common errors that are made in research reports: (a) including too many quotes to represent one point or idea when only a couple of quotes would suffice, (b) presenting a quote without any guidance for the readers regarding what they are reading that quote for, and (c) not appropriately introducing a quote. Qualitative researchers also need to be careful when quoting participants if their actual words can reveal just who they are. This leads into the next topic of publishing qualitative research, namely, the ethics of protecting participants' confidentiality.

The typical small sample size used in qualitative studies can be problematic in that participants could be recognized. Some techniques are available to help resolve the issues of confidentiality in writing qualitative research for publication. One technique involves omitting or changing details about participants to help disguise who they are, for instance, changing demographic variables that have little or no bearing on the results. For example, in my Internet studies of traumatic childbirth, I would change the spelling of some words the mothers used to protect confidentiality. If a mother was from New Zealand, I would change "behaviour" to "behavior." At other times, if a mother had given birth to a son, I may have changed this to a daughter.

Another strategy for presenting qualitative findings is the use of a metaphor. Richardson (1994), in her informative chapter on "Writing: A method of inquiry," introduced metaphor this way:

> A literary device, metaphor is the backbone of social science writing. Like the spine, it bears weight, permits movement, is buried beneath the surface, and links parts together into a functional coherent whole. As this metaphor about metaphor suggests, the essence of metaphor is the experiencing and understanding of one thing in terms of another. This is accomplished through comparison. (p. 519)

If you do decide to use a metaphor, you must take it seriously. Becker (1986) warned that a frequent problem in qualitative research is that authors do not follow through on the details of their metaphor, nor do they carry it throughout the analysis and interpretation. A metaphor needs to be woven throughout the results. Mixing metaphors or using metaphors that do not fit the data are other types of misuse of metaphors (Sandelowski, 1998). Carpenter (2008) cautioned that "misuse of metaphors can create an inaccurate portrayal, casting shadows on the experiences re-presented in the data" (p. 279). Depending on your choice of metaphor, there is a risk that you can oversimplify the phenomenon under study and depict a complex phenomenon as trite (Donovan & Mercer, 2003).

MIXED-METHODS RESEARCH

Writing up a mixed-methods study can be a daunting task (Leech, 2012). Researchers face a number of challenges due to the complexity of this type of study. Researchers need to bring together the results and not treat the qualitative and quantitative strands as separate domains. Writing the report so that it meets the page limitations of a selected journal is a feat in itself. You have to write up all the phases of not only the quantitative strand but also the qualitative strand. For example, you need to describe the quantitative data collection and analysis in addition to the qualitative data collection and analysis.

Leech, Onwuegbuzie, and Combs (2011) identified five challenges of writing mixed-methods research:

1. Writing for a varied audience: both qualitative and quantitative readers
2. Knowing what language to use: qualitative and quantitative terms
3. Having adequate knowledge of both qualitative and quantitative research content
4. Formatting the sections of the report
5. Finding publishing outlets for mixed-methods research studies

From the very start of the manuscript, researchers need to be explicit about the strategies used for each strand of their mixed-methods study at each stage. "Mixed methods" should be in the title of the article. In the introduction of the article, the researcher needs to clearly state the "mixed goal of the study, the mixed research objective(s), the rationale of the study and the rationale(s) for mixing quantitative and qualitative approaches, the purpose of the study and the purpose(s) of mixing quantitative and qualitative approaches, and the mixed research question(s)" (Leech et al., 2011, p. 12). Also, in this first section, the paradigm and theoretical framework, and/or the philosophical perspective that underpins the study need to be clearly stated.

In the next section of the manuscript, the methods section is the focus. The type of sampling and sample size for each strand of the mixed-methods research need to be clearly delineated. Also, the specific mixed-methods research design used, such as a concurrent design, is described along with letting the reader know whether both strands were equal or one was the dominant strand. All of this is necessary to ensure transparency of your methods for the readers.

The third part of the manuscript focuses on research implementation, data collection and analysis, and data interpretation for each strand. When and how were the results integrated? This needs to be clearly explained as well as if the qualitative data were quantitized or the quantitative data qualitized. Specifically address how the use of a mixed-methods approach contributed to the increased understanding of the results.

In each segment of your mixed-methods report, your writing needs to be symmetrical. For instance, if in describing your sampling strategies you first described the quantitative strand followed by the qualitative strand, then keep this order throughout the rest of the manuscript. When you move on to the description of data collection, stay with the format of explaining the quantitative strand before the qualitative strand.

A diagram of your mixed-methods research design is an excellent addition to your manuscript. Visually, a diagram can succinctly and clearly summarize your complex design. In Figure 7.6 is an example of one such diagram from my mixed-methods study on secondary traumatic stress in certified nurse-midwives (Beck, LoGiudice, & Gable, 2015).

Creswell (2015) has developed a checklist of the following elements to include in a mixed-methods manuscript submission:

- Include a mixed-methods title
- Add an abstract that conveys the type of mixed-methods design used
- Convey how the problem merits a mixed-methods study (rationale)
- Create a mixed-methods study aim or purpose statement
- Create quantitative, qualitative, and mixed-methods research questions
- Consider stating the worldview underlying the research and the use of theory (social science, transformative)
- Include rigorous mixed-methods components
  - Discuss the advantages of using mixed-methods
  - Identify the type of mixed-methods design used
  - Present a diagram of procedures
  - Identify methodological challenges
  - Describe quantitative and qualitative data collection and analysis
  - Discuss ethical issues
  - Discuss validity
- Report the results in a manner consistent with the mixed-methods design
- Discuss the integration of quantitative and qualitative data (p. 97)

AVOIDING DUPLICATE PUBLICATION

Obviously, in a program of research and the quest for promotion and tenure in academia, publications are worth their weight in gold. Authors need to avoid duplicate publication, which is "the republication of an article (or a thinly disguised version of an article) in a second journal, without acknowledgment of, or without obtaining permission from, the copyright holder of the first journal" (Morse, 2007, p. 1307). Redundant publication is often referred to as the "salami slicer syndrome," where researchers try to divide up their results from one study into as many publications as possible (Hegyvary, 2005). Pressure to "publish or perish" can drive this practice.

Researchers will have the results of their study to share, but they may also have methodological strategies. One is the conventional report of the

• **FIGURE 7.6 Diagram of the Convergent Parallel Design**

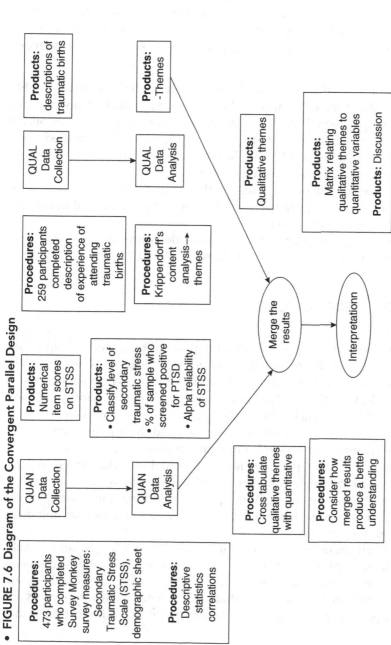

Reprinted with permission from Beck, LoGiudice, & Gable (2015, p.18).

study's results, and the other is a methods article. Sandelowski (2006) gave the following sage advice for anyone planning to publish a methods article before the report of the research results: An author needs to avoid providing more of the results in the first methods article than is necessary because that would make it more difficult to avoid duplication in the secondary article.

Janice Morse, editor of *Qualitative Health Research*, identified several actions that an author is responsible for if publishing from one study in several journals:

1. When submitting the second and subsequent articles for review, notify the editor about the other articles that have been published, are in press, or are in preparation. Because editors are also concerned about duplicate publication, summarize each article in your letter (or if requested, send copies) so the editor may be satisfied that the new article is unique, and that duplicate publication has not occurred.
2. In the acknowledgment footnote, cite the original grant, project, and/or other articles derived from the same data set so that readers, if interested, may easily locate those articles.
3. If the article is a report or translation, provide appropriate attribution to the original article and publisher. (Morse, 2007, p. 1308)

DECIDING WHERE TO PUBLISH

Periodically, there are articles published that are of tremendous help to authors in making the important decision of which journal to submit their manuscript. Northam, Yarbrough, Haas, and Duke (2010) provided one such valuable article, with the title "Journal editor survey: Information to help authors publish." In the article, the results of a survey of 63 journal editors are reported with important journal characteristics and the top three reasons for rejection of manuscripts. Examples of some of these journal characteristics that Northam et al. (2010) provided for each journal included time from submission to decision, article word limit, and percentage of solicited articles. Some of the common reasons editors gave for rejecting a manuscript were that it was poorly written, the topic was not relevant to the journal, and there were methodology problems.

Journal characteristics can certainly help in deciding where to submit your manuscript for publication. You always want to submit to a peer-reviewed journal, but once you have decided which journal, there are other considerations. For example, what audience do you want to read your article—academics or clinicians? Circulation of a journal is important so that you have the largest number of people reading your article. How many issues a year are published? It may take longer to see your article in print if you choose a journal that has only four issues per year versus one that publishes every month. The impact factor is a metric of how often articles in a specific journal have been cited in a particular year. The *Journal of Citation Reports* publishes the impact factors of journals each year. The impact factor is controversial, but deserves some consideration in your journal choice. If you are going to submit a mixed-methods study for publication, you need to consider that there are a few journals that publish only mixed-methods research. These journals include the *Journal of Mixed Methods Research, International Journal of Multiple Research Approaches, Field Methods,* and *Quality and Quantity.*

When you have a short list of journals to which you are considering submitting your manuscript, it is a good idea to look over the table of contents from the past year for each journal to see the topics of articles that have been published. If too many articles have recently been published on the topic of your manuscript in a journal, the editor may not want to publish yet another one on the same topic so soon.

The average time from submission of a manuscript until a decision on publication is very important. A couple of journals took well over one year to decide on whether to accept, revise and resubmit, or reject my manuscript. I will never submit to those journals again. We all know that data get old. Our data-based manuscripts need to be published as soon as possible. All of my articles on my research on traumatic childbirth have been published in *Nursing Research.* This journal's turnaround time is excellent. For illustration purposes, I will share the timeline for the publication of my study entitled "Subsequent Childbirth After a Previous Traumatic Birth" (Beck & Watson, 2010):

> August 17, 2009: Submitted my manuscript to *Nursing Research*
> October 13, 2009: Received a decision of Revise and Resubmit
> December 18, 2009: Submitted my revised manuscript to *Nursing Research*
> January 27, 2010: Manuscript accepted
> July/August 2010: Article published in *Nursing Research*

It took less than 2 months to get the editor's decision of Revise and Resubmit. Once I resubmitted my revised manuscript, it took just a little over 1 month for the revised manuscript to be accepted for publication in *Nursing Research,* and that even included the holidays in that short period. The article was published 5 months later. The online version was even sooner than July.

REFERENCES

American Educational Research Association. (2006). Standards for reporting on empirical social science research in AERA publications. *Educational Researchers, 35,* 33–40.

American Psychological Association. (2010). *Publication manual of the American Psychological Association* (6th ed.). Washington, DC: Author.

Beck, C. T. (1993). Teetering on the edge: A substantive theory of postpartum depression. *Nursing Research, 42*(10), 42–48.

Beck, C. T. (2004a). Post-traumatic stress disorder due to childbirth: The aftermath. *Nursing Research, 53*(4), 216–224.

Beck, C. T. (2004b). Birth trauma: In the eye of the beholder. *Nursing Research, 53,* 28–35.

Beck, C. T. (2006). The anniversary of birth trauma: Failure to rescue. *Nursing Research, 55*(6), 381–390.

Beck, C. T., LoGiudice, J., & Gable, R. K. (2015). Shaken belief in the birth process: A mixed methods study of secondary traumatic stress in certified nurse-midwives. *Journal of Midwifery & Women's Health, 60,* 16–23.

Beck, C. T., & Watson, S. (2008). Impact of birth trauma on breast-feeding: A tale of two pathways. *Nursing Research, 57*(4), 228–236.

Beck, C. T., & Watson, S. (2010). Subsequent childbirth after a previous traumatic birth. *Nursing Research, 59*(4), 241–249.

Becker, H. S. (1986). *Writing for social scientists: How to start and finish your thesis, book, or article.* Chicago, IL: University of Chicago Press.

Carpenter, J. (2008). Metaphors in qualitative research: Shedding light or casting shadows? *Research in Nursing & Health, 31,* 274–282.

Colaizzi, P. F. (1978). Psychological research as the phenomenologist views it. In R. Valle & M. King (Eds.), *Existential phenomenological alternatives for psychology* (pp. 48–71). New York, NY: Oxford University Press.

Creswell, J. W. (2015). *A concise introduction to mixed methods research.* Los Angeles, CA: SAGE.

Donovan, T., & Mercer, D. (2003). Onward in my journey: Preparing nurses for a new age of cancer care. *Cancer Nursing, 26,* 400–404.

Eisner, E. (1998). *The enlightened eye: Qualitative inquiry and the enhancement of educational practice.* Upper Saddle River, NJ: Merril.

Hegyvary, S. T. (2005). What every author should know about redundant and duplicate publication. *Journal of Nursing Scholarship, 37*(4), 295–297.

Leech, N. L. (2012). Writing mixed research reports. *American Behavioral Scientist, 56,* 866–881.

Leech, N. L., Onwuegbuzie, A. J., & Combs, J. P. (2011). Writing publishable mixed research articles: Guidelines for emerging scholars in the health sciences and beyond. *International Journal of Multiple Research Approaches, 5,* 7–24.

Morse, J. M. (2007). Duplicate publication. *Qualitative Health Research, 17*(1), 1307–1308.

Northam, S., Yarbrough, S., Haas, B., & Duke, G. (2010). Journal editor survey: Information to help authors publish. *Nurse Educator, 35*(1), 29–36.

Richardson, L. (1994). Writing: A method of inquiry. In N. K. Denzin & Y. S. Lincoln (Eds.), *Handbook of qualitative research* (pp. 516–529). Thousand Oaks, CA: SAGE.

Sandelowski, M. (1994). The use of quotes in qualitative research. *Research in Nursing & Health, 17,* 479–482.

Sandelowski, M. (1998). Writing a good read: Strategies for re–presenting qualitative data. *Research in Nursing & Health, 21,* 375–382.

Sandelowski, M. (2003). Tables or tableaux? The challenges of writing and reading mixed methods studies. In A. Tashakkori & C. Teddlie (Eds.), *Handbooks of mixed methods in social and behavioral sciences.* Thousand Oaks, CA: SAGE.

Sandelowski, M. (2006). Divide and conquer: Avoiding duplication in the reporting of qualitative research. *Research in Nursing & Health, 29,* 371–373.

Van Manen, M. (2002). *Writing in the dark: Phenomenological studies in interpretive inquiry.* London, Ontario, Canada: The Althouse Press.

Epilogue

Throughout this book, I have used the metaphor of paths to illustrate points I have made regarding the evolution of a successful research trajectory. It is my hope that after reading this book, when you are at each crossroad in your research program deciding on your next study, you will not immediately choose the trodden path, the beaten path that keeps that path "a sacred groove." A researcher's choice of path leads to other forks in the road and so on. You, as the researcher, may never have the chance to go back to travel that road not taken.

In the discipline of nursing, our patients are so complex that the research conducted to provide the best evidence-based practice needs to include both quantitative and qualitative research. The progression of the most valuable research programs is knowledge driven and not method limited. Examples from my 25-year program of research on postpartum mood and anxiety disorders have been used to illustrate the main ideas in each chapter. Armed with the "tools and materials" presented here, you can design a research program that invites nurses and other health care providers to "linger and stroll" there in order to provide them with valuable evidence to apply in their clinical practice. Numerous books have been published for years on how to write successful grants, but until now a book devoted to demonstrating how to develop a successful program of research was lacking.

Index

Printed in the United States
By Bookmasters